Finley's Footprints
Mel Scott

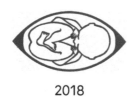

2018

Finley's Footprints

Mel Scott

August 2018 (1.4)

ISBN 978-1-908293-48-0

Published by:

Birthing Awareness

An imprint of CGW Publishing
B 1502
PO Box 15113
Birmingham
B2 2NJ
United Kingdom

www.birthingawareness.com

www.towards-tomorrow.com

www.finleysfootprints.com

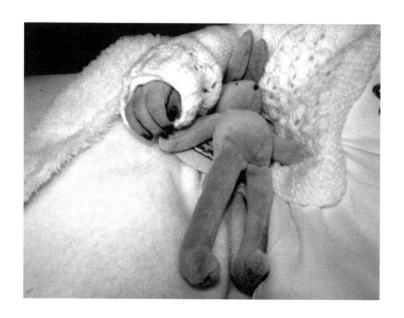

I held an angel in my arms; he left his footprints in my heart.

For Finley – always for Finley.

Foreword

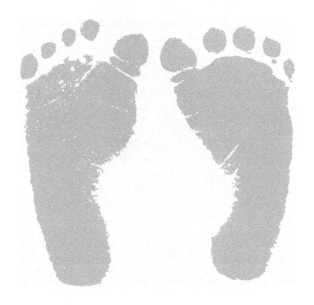

Finley's Footprints was written by a mother who, sadly, has loved and lost two babies. The first was lost by miscarriage on the day after Mother's Day, March 2008. The baby did not make it to eight weeks' gestation, and was never named or buried. Despite this, the mother thinks of this baby as a baby. She had imagined all the things they would do together, and the baby is thought about and missed to this day. The second baby lost was Finley. A beautiful baby boy, Finley was born sleeping at six thirteen in the morning of Sunday, August 2nd 2009 after forty-one weeks and five days of a perfect pregnancy. After forty-one weeks and five days of planning, hoping and dreaming that this time things would be different.

Finley's Footprints is the moving story of a heartbroken yet resilient young family's day-to-day life in the shadow of grief. In its highly readable account of the intricate, often mundane details of everyday life after loss, the book casts taboos aside and faces grief head on, confounding expectations and challenging fears. In the process, it brings to light vital insights into the needs of parents of stillborn babies (as well as babies lost through miscarriage or other medical complications). It also makes clear the ways in which family, friends, healthcare practitioners and other related professionals can make a difference. Everyone including midwives, health visitors, doctors and consultants, vicars, chaplains and other religious officiators and funeral directors will find something in this book to answer their questions or help improve their understanding. Anyone who has experienced or is currently experiencing a loss will, hopefully, find suggestions here that help them survive it.

Finley's Footprints is also a love story. The story of one woman's discovery of a love so powerful and expansive that it transcends even death. The story of her journey from suffering to acceptance and peace. In it, the author discusses how she learnt to connect with the peace within her, and so discovered the means to express herself fully and authentically in the world. What you might call a 'spiritual' journey but if it is, it's neither religious nor preachy, and it's certainly never conventional. It's an honest, hopeful and compelling story with a liberal scattering of irreverent humour. Finley's Footprints is a book that could convince even the most sceptical reader of the power of love to transform the life we live and the lives of those around us. The author believes that every person – every soul – has a purpose. It's just that this purpose is only ever likely to be revealed in the most unexpected ways.

There are many ways in which Finley's life has made a difference in the world; chief among them is the existence of registered charity Towards Tomorrow Together, established in Finley's memory and in memory of all 'angel babies' to offer supportive services for parents experiencing the loss of a baby. The author also runs Finley's Footprints, which provides a range of coaching and training services for parents and professionals who find their lives touched by the loss of a baby. You'll find further information about these organisations and the services they offer at the end of this book (see the Afterword on page 288) as well as online at www.towards-tomorrow.com and www.finleysfootprints.com.

A dream

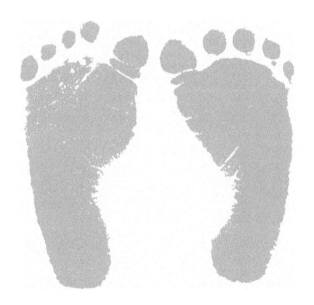

There is a place on top of the hills where we go for walks. It is an incredibly beautiful spot, peaceful and wild. From here, you can see for miles in every direction: down into the valley to my parents' place and the town where we live, then right out as far as the sea. On a clear day, you can even set eyes on Wales. It's usually pretty blustery up here, and really blows away the cobwebs. Right at the summit stands a circle of three ancient oak trees, all that now remain of the original Seven Sisters.

I hear a dreamy sound that fills my heart with joy. It's coming from behind the circle of oaks. I move towards the enchanting melody, and catch a glimpse of a little boy chasing his sister across the clearing and down the side of the hill. She is giggling and screaming, running as fast as her little legs can carry her. I watch as they both run through ferns so tall that all I can see is their heads bobbing among the colourful flowers.

The girl is around four and the boy maybe a year or so younger. I can tell that he has blue eyes, shining brightly just like his mum's. The girl is blessed to have inherited her dad's olive skin tone and deep, dark brown eyes. The two children look so much alike, as each one's angelic blonde curls are tossed about in the breeze.

I run after the children, calling out to them to wait for me. But as I reach the brow of the hill, expecting to see them just over the other side, they have disappeared. I am left with the sound of my dream as it dies on the breeze. My heart breaks once again.

Prologue

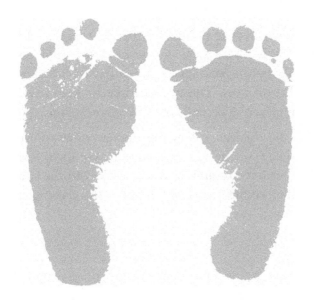

In the first few days after my son Finley was born, I started writing a journal. My husband Baz and I had just come home from hospital without our baby. We had left him with virtual strangers to face the ordeal of a post-mortem alone. The jumbled mess of thoughts raging in my mind was unbearable. At first, I wrote simply to get the thoughts out of my head. I wrote in the hope that I might rest. But after a while, when I started to read back over what I'd written, I saw that what I had to say could be useful. I saw that my memories could help others if I had the means to turn the journal into a book. Other parents who had lost a baby would find a point of reference for their own experiences as well as all sorts of vital information. Perhaps some comfort to know they are not alone. Professionals working with bereaved parents would see how influential their care can be. They would gain a deeper understanding of the small things they can do to change a parent's life forever.

My journal entries begin five days after Finley was born and end the day, more than three months later, when we received the results of his post-mortem examination. In my journal, I record the intimate experiences of those early, difficult days after his death.[i] I talk about all those details and everyday tasks, decisions, conversations and thoughts that, in the face of grief, can seem so utterly insurmountable. After several days of writing, I also found myself composing little notes to Finley at the end of each day's journal entry. I'd found a way I could communicate with my son, talk to him and tell him I loved him. Over time, these notes to Finley started to tell their own story. One in which the experience of grief opens into a love so unifying and expansive that it changed my world and everything I believed to be true.

Although Finley's Footprints covers only the few months after Finley was born, it is also the story of the start of the rest of our lives. My son Finley may have died, but this memoir lives on. Here it is at last, the story of a love a zillion times bigger than the sky.

* * *

Before my journal of the period after Finley can begin, I want to tell you about our time with Finley. A time that begins right back before he was even conceived.

In March 2008, I had a miscarriage. It had been my first pregnancy. My husband Baz and I had planned for it and had been trying for a few months. I discovered I was pregnant at the same time as my friend Jade. Less than a week later, I began to bleed.

I went to hospital and there my roller-coaster journey began. I was told I had made a mistake with my dates. The scan showed just an egg sac. I had a blood test and was asked to come back for a further test to check my hormone levels. The levels hadn't doubled as they should have done, so the doctors wanted to test me for a different hormone. If the levels of this hormone were high enough, then the pregnancy would be viable. But the levels were found to be inadequate to support a pregnancy and we were told we would lose the baby.

It took almost a week before the miscarriage actually happened. During that week, I continued at work as if nothing was wrong. I felt completely let down by the professionals. I'd been treated as though there was nothing going on here but a medical incident. Nobody seemed to think that this was a baby. Except me.

After a few weeks' rest, I tried to get on with my life. I remember very clearly a dream I had at the time. A baby girl was lying on a fern bed, the sunlight catching her skin and sparkling. She was holding her feet with her hands in that cute way only babies can, and gurgling and giggling to herself. I knew this was the baby I had lost, and was able to say thank you to her. And goodbye.

I thought I had recovered quite well, until it got close to the day my baby would have been due. Jade had her baby on that exact same day. I was delighted for her – she gave birth to a beautiful baby boy. But I was devastated for us. Suddenly, I realised how important it had become to me to be a mum. Baz and I visited Jade in hospital and she was fantastic: the minute I arrived she handed baby Harvey to me, and left the room. I sat there hugging her baby, crying and sobbing. When we left the hospital, I told Baz I wanted us to stop trying for a baby. I couldn't handle the heartache every month. Two weeks later I discovered I was pregnant.

Around this time, I went to see a psychic. She mentioned that she felt a spirit close to me, just behind me and to my left. She sensed it was a wise, calm spirit. I had no idea who or what this spirit could be, so put it to the back of my mind. I didn't know then, but this presence behind me and to the left would soon reappear.

I was delighted to discover I was pregnant again. In fact, something happened to me during the early part of my pregnancy. I found a deep sense of peace. Once I'd got past the twelve weeks milestone, I happily assumed everything would go smoothly. I never considered the possibility that something could happen later on. Getting pregnant and carrying a healthy baby to term should be easy. I mean, it's the most natural thing in the world, isn't it?

My friend Carolyn gave me a book called The Gentle Birth Method. It was exactly the right thing to help me to nurture myself and my baby. I followed the advice which included listening to birth preparation relaxation exercises daily, frequent walking and swimming, and taking good care over my diet. Most of all, I enjoyed the required pampering – finally someone had given me permission to treat myself. I had regular Reiki and reflexology treatments. The baby seemed to enjoy the Reiki especially, and would wake up and move around in a very distinct way – gently and serenely – under the therapist's hands. When the baby and I connected with one another during this time (my mind connecting with the baby's soul it seemed), I felt the sensation that my baby was behind and to the left of me. I also felt quite clearly that this baby was a very wise, old soul and not the new soul I had expected.

The baby got into the correct position, but nothing else happened. My due date came and went and there were still no signs of labour. So I was promptly booked in for an induction. I was extremely disappointed to think that I had got this close to having a natural birth and yet now it would have to be medicalised. I so desperately wanted a water birth with just a tens machine as pain relief in the early stages. I wanted the birth to be peaceful. So, I began in earnest trying everything to move this baby along. We must have eaten curry ten times in a single week. Then I had an acupuncture treatment that seemed to start some contractions, so I carried on using the acupressure points and taking the recommended homeopathic remedies.

Three days before I was scheduled to have the induction, I thought my waters had broken. I phoned the hospital and they suggested I come in to be checked. I was so relaxed about it all that I asked them if it was alright for me to stay home and watch Casualty first. We got to the hospital at ten on the Saturday night. The midwife told us there was meconium in the waters. They wanted to put me on a monitor. I was worried and asked about my water birth. I wouldn't be able to go ahead with it. I was so upset I cried and threatened to go home. They checked the baby's heartbeat on the monitor and, because it was strong, advised me to stay in overnight and settle myself onto the ward. As I was not in established labour, Baz was sent home. When the midwife did an internal to start things off, she told me my cervix had not changed and I was still in early labour. Although I was having contractions, I could not feel them.

All seemed well and I settled down to try and relax as much as I could, given that I hadn't wanted to be in hospital. I listened to my relaxation CD over and over again, and continued using the homeopathic remedies and pushing on the acupressure points. Then, at four in the morning, the midwife checked the monitor and I told her the numbers indicated that the baby's heartbeat kept on dropping. I got worried because the meconium had clearly got thicker as well. After keeping an eye on the monitor for a while, the midwife called someone else to check it out. The baby had gone into distress. A doctor carried out an ultrasound and found that the baby's heartbeat was too slow. An emergency caesarean section took place at five fifty-five in the morning. Yet there was still nothing in the attitude of the staff to suggest anything was wrong with the baby.

I don't remember much after that. I think I phoned Baz and asked him to come back. I was taken into the operating theatre. I remember a foul-smelling mask being plastered over my face and someone pushing down on my throat. I fell asleep with tears rolling down my cheeks. I think I knew my baby had gone.

Looking back, I had never been able to imagine leaving the hospital with a baby, or bringing a baby home. I had visualised the birth, but never further into the future than that. Maybe I was never meant to bring my baby home. It's easy to over-analyse things with the benefit of hindsight. And too easy to blame myself.

Our little boy Finley was born at thirteen minutes past six on the morning of Sunday, August 2nd 2009. He was born without a heartbeat. In the eighteen minutes it had taken for the doctors to decide to operate, anaesthetise me and carry out a caesarean, my baby had been born. He had been born but he did not wake up.

I don't think I took it in when they told me. I vaguely recall screaming No!, but I don't really remember much of anything. I'd been given a lot of morphine. I know Mum gave me Finley to hold, but I must have fallen asleep again. I have photographs of that first morning, not memories. There are photos of Mum holding Finley, as well as of Beverley (Baz's mum) and her partner Mick. I know that Jade and Ross visited too (Jade had brought proper tissues with her). I think my brother Stephen and his girlfriend Denise may have come, but we don't have any photos of them there. My friends Katy and Roger were with us at some point, and I know I made a couple of phone calls, but I have little memory of any of them. What could I have said when my beautiful baby boy had been born but would remain asleep forever?

Baz arrived too late to see his son born. What it was like for him to have rushed to get there and then arrive to hear such news, I'll never be able to imagine. He did so well. He phoned everyone in the one morning. How he managed it, or what he told people, I honestly don't know. I'm just so grateful he was able to do this for us. Eventually, I think Baz had someone with him, babysitting him, making sure he was okay. I am glad.

On the Sunday, I was moved into the Conway Suite, the bereavement room just down the corridor from the main labour ward. Any mother who loses a baby at more than sixteen weeks' gestation – whether before, during or shortly after birth – is cared for here. It's a small room, decked out to be more homely than a hospital room. It has a divan bed with a quilt rather than the usual hospital sheets and blankets. There's a candle ornament and a television in there, as well as a small en suite bathroom.

I think I held Finley that evening, and remember ringing the bell to get the midwife to put him in his cot to sleep. At that stage, I don't think any of it felt real at all. Perhaps some part of me knew he was dead, but another part simply wasn't going to let that be a reality. Finley slept in his cot at the end of my bed. There are photos of him in a Moses basket, so I'm not sure when they exchanged that for the cot. Still, I remember being pleased as punch that he had a cot like all the other babies did.

By Monday I was in pain. The morphine dose was stopped and I was told I'd have to go home. It's the only time I remember anyone saying we would have to leave the hospital. I didn't want to leave. No one had said it outright, but I knew that when we left we wouldn't be taking Finley with us.

I tried to have a shower after they removed the morphine wires. I remember being in tears in the bathroom, standing on one leg trying to get into the bath. No one had told me that when I stood up I would bleed heavily. Because of my stitches I couldn't even reach the floor to clean up. I was sobbing my heart out and remember shouting at the poor midwife. It seemed so unfair to be in physical pain when I had no baby. If I had a fucking baby to look after I wouldn't want any painkillers! I yelled. But I don't have a baby! The midwife was gentle, explaining that the emotional pain was making the physical pain worse. Still, I got more medication in the end.

My friends Alana and Bianca visited. Bianca held Finley and it meant the world to me. Watching my friends meet my little boy seemed to validate his life. To prove that he was real and that he did exist. Alana brought Finley a little rabbit and it was like a weight lifted from me. I'd been desperately upset that nobody had bought Finley presents. All we had were cards and flowers. Now of course, I feel ungrateful, but at the time I just wanted Finley to have his presents. Maybe it was a need to celebrate his birth. But perhaps more simply, if people bought gifts it helped me believe that Finley was sleeping in his cot just like any other baby.

Baz's dad Tony and his girlfriend Liz visited as well. Liz had experienced a stillbirth in the family last year, so it seemed to help her a lot when she held Finley, even though it must have been difficult, rekindling sad memories. Amid all the visitors, I remember hearing the frustrated midwife telling me I needed to rest. I was angry and said I'd have lots of time to rest soon. After all I had no baby to look after.

By this point, I had discovered that I loved cuddling Finley and I would not let him go. That night, Baz stayed with the two of us in the little room. Our one precious night together as a family.

On Tuesday, Baz went home to collect some bits and pieces for Finley. I suspect he was pretty fed up by this stage. I'd made him take almost a hundred photos. Still, he came back with a whole pile of outfits we'd bought especially for Finley. He also brought in a Winnie-the-Pooh teddy bear. We dressed Finley in all the different outfits – a kind of fashion show – and took photos of him wearing them. I have the teddy bear now at home in Finley's cot. It's precious because Finley had it with him in hospital and, later, took it with him to the post-mortem.

Baz did not stay with us the Tuesday night. He needed sleep. At some point a decision was made that we would go home the following day. I don't know how, or who had decided. Jill, the bereavement midwife, spent a long time with me that night since I couldn't sleep. She persuaded me to think carefully about what I wanted my last memory of Finley to be. She took time out to prepare me – all the time I needed. I realised very clearly that all we had left to us was a very short space of time in which to make the only memories of Finley we'd have, and be able to keep for the rest of our lives. I spent that night holding Finley, cuddling up to him. Sleeping with my baby in my arms. We took photos of the two of us. You can see my tears in them. Even though they're distressing, the memories are precious. I wouldn't be without them. For me, there's nothing more beautiful – more natural – than a mum cradling her baby as he sleeps.

At some point during the night, I think Finley's soul left his body. At the time, I didn't understand what I was feeling, but with hindsight, there was definitely a point when Finley left his body behind. Up until that moment I had stayed connected to Finley through his body. This was different to the connection we'd shared when he was actually inside me. When he'd been in my womb, I'd sensed him as a presence outside of me, behind me and to the left. But when we were in hospital, the focus of our connection quickly became this tiny, vulnerable little body in my arms, or snuggled in his cot. All this changed overnight.

On the morning of the last day I felt absolutely certain that Finley was not in his body any more. Perhaps this was the process of me coming to realise fully that our baby was dead. But he was still present in the room. I could feel quite distinctly the love and peace that I know is Finley. Right there in the room but now detached from my baby's body. Some days later, I had the privilege to connect with Finley's soul again, on the night we brought him home. I cannot explain any of this more precisely, nor do I ask you to believe me. I'm simply stating the truth as I experienced it.

In total we were able to spend three days in hospital with Finley. I will be forever thankful for this – most people in our situation don't get anything like this long. But eventually we had to leave. And we did so in a whirl of emotion. For much of the time, we were numb to the whole thing and just going through the motions. I had decided that I wanted my last memory of Finley to be bathing him, dressing him and reading him a story before leaving him in that cosy room with a midwife so he would not be alone. We now have special videos of these moments. They are the most extraordinary and moving videos I have ever seen. A mum caring for her baby, changing his nappy, washing him and getting the poppers done up all wrong. Then cuddling him as she reads him a bedtime story, wraps him in a blanket and lays him in his cot to sleep. It looks like the most natural thing in the world. Until you realise the baby's lips are black and he is all floppy. Until you realise that this baby will not wake up the next morning. That his parents will never feel his breath on their cheeks. That they'll never grumble as they hear him cry at three in the morning. That they'll never see what colour his eyes are, or know the sound of his cry.

The one thing they will remember, for the rest of their lives, is walking down that corridor accompanied by the sound of other babies crying, and knowing that they are walking away from their baby for the last time.

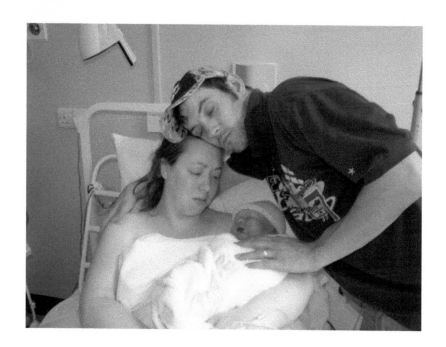

If we could have a lifetime wish

A dream that would come true

We'd pray to God with all our hearts

For yesterday and you.

A thousand words can't bring you back

We know because we've tried

Neither will a thousand tears

We know because we've cried.

You left behind our broken hearts

And happy memories too

We never wanted memories

We only wanted you

Unknown author

Day 5

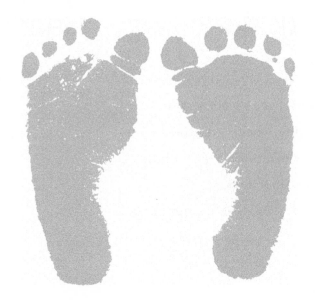

I am not sure how to start. Or what the point of writing is. I don't know why I feel I need to put things down on paper. Perhaps it's enough that it'll give me something to do. Help me get through these long days. Give me a distraction.

Maybe it will help me remember what has happened. Hold on to precious memories. I am so worried I will forget him. It seems too easy to forget. To move on. As if he was never here.

I guess it's finger-to-key. Form a letter, then a word, then a page. One step at a time, just as we're getting through life right now. One meal. One sleep. One minute. One hour. One day at a time.

Today is the first day I have felt part of this world again. I've had some tearful moments, but also more positive ones. I may even have smiled. Our midwife – the lovely Barb – visited us today. She said this is not the way it was supposed to be.

Barb gave us a card with Baby Boy on the front. It's the first card we've received celebrating a birth, rather than saying thinking of you. It's important that someone recognises he was here. That he came to us and was part of this family.

Barb and I looked through hundreds of photos together. I cried again this time. He looks as if he will wake up at any minute, as if he is sleeping in my arms. Barb commented on his chubby cheeks, saying he's a big lad. Bigger than she thought he'd be.

A friend came to see me. She was lovely, and looked through our photos too. She had lost a baby when she was younger, it must have been difficult for her. She told me how important it is to stay with your feelings, not to block them out. She said if you block them out you'll have to deal with them later. It's a lesson I've been learning over and over these past few years. In fact, my friend Tania has commented on how present I am to all my feelings. I am just in them, she said.

The computer broke down, and I feel lost and isolated. I can't imagine not being able to go on Facebook. People there have been such a comfort. I hope a friend will be able to fix the computer.

It is the post-mortem today. I can only hope they find out what happened to our baby boy. He is so far away in Bristol. I just want him to be here with us.

Day 6

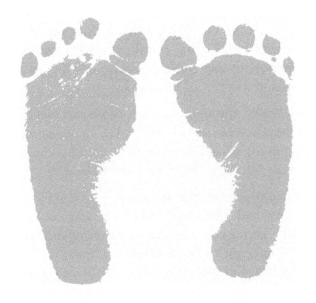

I woke in the night after a bad dream of a tall man with curly hair in a white medical jacket standing at the bottom of my bed. I say bad dream: maybe it wasn't, it didn't frighten me. I just felt incredibly lonely and cried.

It's funny how much closer he seems at night. Gizmo (our ginger cat) came onto the bed for a cuddle, which helped fill the huge gap in my arms. But he's not the right shape to fill the space my baby has left behind.

I spent a lot of the day asleep on the sofa. Mum visited in the afternoon. Bless her, she's taken some of our washing home with her. She came with a set of photos taken on her camera, and helped me put them into an album. There's one of my dad sitting next to my son at the head of the cot. We don't have many of the two of them: Dad found it hard to be there, his grandson looking as if he could so easily just wake up.

I'm still not sure which tense I should be writing in. Past or present? In a way, either is right, since it feels like he's still here with me. I guess it doesn't matter.

Lots of Mum's photos were taken while I was still asleep: I'd had a general anaesthetic, so I think I slept most of the Sunday. We took our photos later on, and I hadn't seen Mum's until now. I don't remember much at all from the day he was born.

Mum brought us a card and a little grey baby-boy bear in a baby-boy gift bag. On the card, there's a picture of a grey bear asleep in baby-boy clothes. Inside, Mum has written his full name. It feels very special when people acknowledge that he was born. I want other people to think of him too. I feel very close to my mum and dad at the moment, which is wonderful.

Leanne, Jason and Matt visited tonight, with a big bottle of vodka. They're close friends of ours from Plymouth and they've been fantastic. Leanne and I used to joke that, since I didn't touch a drop when I was pregnant, as soon as I'd had the baby we'd down an entire bottle of vodka and leave the boys to babysit. She's had that bottle waiting for ages. We all sat down to watch the videos of the first few hours after the birth – mostly videos of Baz bathing and dressing our baby. They laughed at the bit where Baz and the midwife are discussing the fact that he has Baz's ears.

This is especially poignant for me. When I was pregnant, I teased Baz saying I hope the baby has my nose, and we laughed about Baz's mismatched ears (his right is larger than his left). Baz says it's because, when he was young, his mum dragged him home for tea by his right ear. Our son has different sized ears too. But I will never get to drag him home by them.

We also have a video of Jane, the hospital chaplain, giving our son his name. The day after he was born, a midwife had told us we could see Jane. All I knew about hospital chaplains was that they read people their last rites. But we agreed to see her anyway. We would've done anything we were told.

Our son's name is Finley John Scott. Baz chose it while I was pregnant. I'd settled quickly on a name for a girl but Baz took a lot longer to find a boy's name. He's a Liverpool supporter and insisted on trying out every single team member's name. I'd refused point blank to call my baby Gerrard!

At one time I think Baz liked the name Alfie. Then someone told him they knew a little boy called Alfie who was very naughty. So Baz chose the name Finley after seeing an ad on TV for a Finley Quaye album. We had lots of discussions about how to spell the name before settling on Finley rather than Finlay or Finnley. John is both Baz's and my brother's middle name.

It's really hard to watch the video of the service – I look so detached from it all. Finley is in my arms, but I'm not really holding him. Baz is looking down and can hardly look at us. Mum and Dad are there too, and I'm glad they were. Jane explains what she will do and asks us what religion we are. She asks will it be okay to say a prayer and for us all to say the Lord's Prayer together? Then she talks about the Lord God being present in times of sadness and pain, as well as joy and happiness. I remember not wanting to think about God at all – if there is a God, how could he take Finley away from us? Jane says we are angry, scared and mixed up because what should have been a time of joy, excitement and laughter has turned into one of sadness, desolation and misery. It looks as though hearing those words makes me cry, and I start to sob again as I'm watching.

Jane asks God how will we bear it? She says we don't want to give this little one to you. We want to keep him here. But we know we can't do that. We are going to give him his name that Mummy and Daddy have chosen, so they can keep him in their hearts. It's heartbreaking when she says this. She puts a cross on Finley's head, saying he's a beautiful baby. She asks God to receive his soul, welcome him to play with the angels and take care of him until his mummy and daddy can cuddle him again. Then she holds my hand and we all say the Lord's prayer together. The words never seem to make much sense to me. But we finish and Jane asks God to give us the comfort we need. I smile to myself when she gets Baz's name wrong. She calls him Scott. That'd make him Scott Scott no less!

His son died too, Jane says – so God knows something of what we're going through. I start to cry again. It just doesn't make sense. If God knows what we're going through, why would he let us experience this? No one should ever have to go through this.

Baz is being fantastic. He's looking after me. He hates all things medical, but has been giving me injections and sorting out my tablets. He made me laugh earlier, giving me my injection and saying you may feel a little prick. Believe me, giggling while someone tries to stick a needle into you is not a good idea.

Day 7

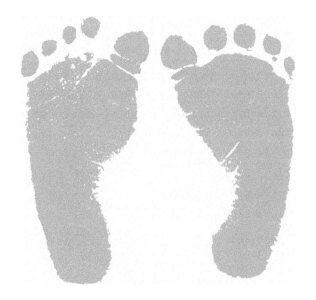

A sad day. Finley should have been one week old. The sun was shining and I could easily imagine walking around with him in his buggy, showing him off. It's hard to believe a week has passed. My life has stopped. Yet time moves on. That's harsh.

I have showered and eaten, and it feels like an achievement. Last night was the first time I've felt hungry. It must've been the vodka.

We went to collect my prescription from the hospital where we'd been for antenatal appointments. Back then, we were full of excitement to hear Finley's heartbeat. I almost wrote your heartbeat. It feels like I'm writing this to Finley. I walked round Sainsbury's afterwards and managed to avoid the baby clothes and toy aisles, only to get to the pharmacy and burst into tears because it's right next to the nappies.

Jade came to visit this afternoon from Cardiff. It was hard and lots of tears were shed. It feels like we've been here before. Like a rerun of a dreadful TV drama. Jade and I were pregnant at the same time last year. It was only when she found out she was pregnant that I realised my period was late. We were so excited to be pregnant together.

Jade gave birth to her baby Harvey the same day our first baby would have been due. At the time, I'd thought that visiting her in hospital after he was born and cuddling him was the hardest thing I'd ever have to do. How wrong I was.

Jade brought with her a box of chocolates from her oldest son, Harry. He wanted them to help us stop feeling sad. Jade also gave me a lavender-scented heat bag in the shape of a cuddly dog. It's funny because right now my arms feel so empty that I just want to hug everything. But it's my baby I long to hold. A heat bag just won't do.

We watched the DVD I've made of all the videos we got taken of Finley. I'm so glad we had that new camera. It was just as painful as it was yesterday to watch the naming ceremony and hear the chaplain's words. But other parts made me smile, such as when Baz bathes his baby boy for the first time, looking so natural as a dad. I laugh now when I remember that Baz had to help me dress Finley because I had no idea what I was doing.

The last scene is the most moving. I'm reading Finley his first — and last — bedtime story. Cradling him in my arms. I'm so grateful to the midwife for encouraging me to think about what I wanted my last memory of Finley to be. She spent a long time helping me explore the things I could do during our last few hours together. It helped me realise that what was upsetting me most was the fact that I'd not done anything personal for my baby. I hadn't washed him, dressed him, fed him or changed his nappy. I hadn't had a chance to do all the normal, everyday things that I long so much to do now. So I decided I wanted to bath him, get him dressed and read to him.

On-screen I'm in tears. I'm reading a story about a baby tiger falling asleep. The other animals can't find him. And, at the end, they say, we missed you baby tiger. I read the words to Finley. Then I kiss him on the little comma-shaped birthmark by his right eyebrow. I wrap him in a blanket and put him in his cot to sleep. I even support his head and put his feet at the bottom of the cot. Just like all the baby books tell you. The most instinctive thing a Mum can do for her baby. The only difference is that I know my beautiful baby boy will not wake up tomorrow. He will never wake up with the sun on his face. I am sobbing as I tell him he can go to sleep now.

Just after this was filmed, we'd walked out of the room and left our baby boy alone with near strangers. Knowing what had happened next made watching the video desperately upsetting. After three days with Finley, I hadn't wanted to go. I hadn't wanted to leave him there.

We'd made the decision the previous day that we'd leave then. I'd talked to Baz that morning about how we'd do it. But he and the midwife still had to support me. I had to try so hard not to look back. One midwife told us that most people in our situation want to leave hospital as soon as they can. But I didn't. I wanted to stay there with my baby forever. I did not want to face the real world outside those doors.

Jade has brought us a memory box she made herself. The box is white, not much bigger than a shoe box. On it is a silver card with Finley's name on, and wrapped around it is a sweet blue ribbon covered in footprints. We're not ready to look at the box yet. So it's on the table, covered up.

I sent an email to a group of friends earlier. We were on a course together last year and they were waiting for news about my baby. I wrote:

Hi,

I am not really sure how to start this email or what to say. I guess the philosophy of taking baby steps that has seen me through my whole spiritual journey will apply here too.

A few weeks ago I was thinking with excitement that I would be able to write with some fantastic news to share. I usually tend to post on this group when I am sad, or need to reach out and feel connected. A few weeks ago I was eagerly and impatiently awaiting the birth of our first baby, much-loved and wanted after the miscarriage last year that shook our whole lives.

On Sunday we had a little baby boy called Finley John. He was nearly two weeks overdue when my waters broke and we trotted off to hospital full of excitement. At 6.13 a.m. on Sunday morning our beautiful baby boy was born by emergency caesarean section. He didn't wake up after his birth. We did not get to hear him cry, or see him take his first feed. He weighs 9 lb 7 oz.

The doctors do not know what happened, and Finley had a post-mortem and lots of tests on Friday. We will not get the results for four months, and the doctors have said that 75% of the time they will not find a reason for something so sudden and unexpected.

Physically, I am not in any pain and am up and moving around remarkably quickly. I know that I am not pregnant any more, but I am struggling a bit with a body that does not feel like mine, a body that feels empty and strange.

Many of you have shared life skills courses with me, or I have assisted on yours. You will have shared my journey through all the hurt and pain of my past, and seen the life I am meant to lead blossom ahead of me. I can honestly say that over the past nine months I have been able to find a rest and a peace that previously I had only dreamed of. I have known true happiness, excitement and joy during a perfect pregnancy, and felt amazingly connected to both Baz and our baby. In some moments I am able to find a path through this, and know that there will be amazing things to come for us; at other moments I am a mummy and have an empty space in my arms, and a heart that feels as if it will burst.

People have been so kind and I am overwhelmed by the cards, flowers and messages. I have had heartfelt messages on Facebook from people I have never met which have reminded me that people are amazing and so kind. It has been a refreshing change to my view of the world which has hurt me in the past.

Everybody has offered to help in any way they can. Those of you who know me will know that I find it very difficult to ask for help, accept help and support or compliments. Much of my journey has been spent learning to allow people to take care of themselves and learning to take care of myself.

I would like to ask anyone who feels able, to support Baz and me through this time ahead. We have lots of things to arrange in the next week before the funeral sometime after 17th August.

If you would like to think of us and send love and light to us, please join us in lighting a candle at the time of the funeral.

Lots of love Mel.

I had three immediate replies. Then a phone call from Tania who said the email had made her cry. She couldn't look at my Facebook page either, as it was too harrowing.

I've searched the internet and found that people refer to babies who've been stillborn as angel babies. Because they're born with wings instead of feet. I asked my friend Carolyn if she'd send me some pictures of angel babies and today I received her email with images of winged babies attached. One is a really cute tattoo. I think I may have it on my back. I'd like to get a tattoo designed from Finley's photograph. And to make a website in his memory too.

Mum phoned to talk about calling the funeral directors. Neither of us know what to expect as we've never had to arrange a funeral before. I had the idea that we could have the service at the church where Baz and I got married. Then food at the Cedar Falls Hotel. We could have the burial just for family later on. That way we'll be able to leave without having to say goodbye to everyone else.

I never, ever thought we would have to think about such things. It's just not fair. Right now we should be tired and excited and holding our baby in our arms. We should be up to our armpits in nappies. Not thinking about hymns and flowers and readings.

On Facebook, my friend Chloë has posted a poem on my wall. Other people seem able to find the words. I want to start writing poems again, but I'm frightened I won't find the right words to express how I feel. Words are not enough. But they are all I have. When will the tears stop? Why can't we wake up, find out this is just a bad dream and that in reality we're still waiting for our precious little baby to arrive?

Day 8

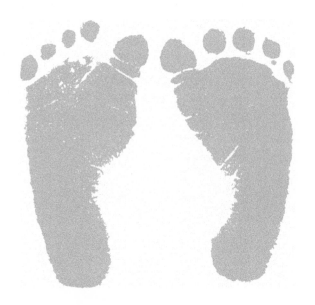

Time has passed so quickly today. I've been busy. It's already eleven and I don't want to miss writing. I've only eaten once and then not even an entire meal. I'm not hungry. Food just doesn't seem important. I've ordered a juicing book online. At least I can get some nutrition that way.

I didn't wake up for my painkillers in the night, and I had no pain, which is great. I've been taking an assortment from the little bag I brought home from the hospital. Some are anti-inflammatories, some reduce the pain from the operation, and the others reduce the side effects of the pain medication. I also have a box full of the injections to prevent blood clots that Baz has been giving me. Still, I am a bit achy. Hardly surprising, since I have been out and about today and sitting at the computer for five hours! Thank goodness the doctors did such a good job of the operation and stitches. The physical scar is really short. It's quite amazing. So much shorter than I'd expected. My tummy is returning to normal very quickly too.

We went to register Finley's birth and death today. It was awful. Not something I thought I would ever have to do. Now we have a certificate. I don't know what to do with it yet. It's so difficult for me to read it. It's not a birth certificate but a Certificate of Stillbirth. Finley was minutes away from being born alive. So close. Would his certificate have been different had he been alive when he was born? Perhaps then he'd have had a birth certificate and a death certificate.

Some of Baz's family visited. Baz spent most of the time playing every conceivable game on the Xbox with his young cousin, Max. Baz's uncle Graham is so upset by what's happened that he doesn't think they'll be able to come to the funeral. Adult funerals upset Graham so much that he just doesn't think he can manage a child's. I remember how distressed he was at Baz's granddad's funeral, so cannot blame him.

I don't want to go to the funeral either. I wonder what would happen if I didn't? It already feels as though it's just something we're obliged to do. Something that's expected of us. Another decision to make. Another part of someone else's process.

We talked about the birth. There are so many similarities with Graham and Carole's daughter Leonie's birth. Leonie has Ataxia Telangiectasia (AT), a very rare genetic condition. While AT appears similar to Cerebral Palsy at first, it worsens over time. Our conversation got me thinking again about whether Finley's death could be related to AT. Carole has already called Ann, the family worker at the AT society, about it. Since Leonie is one of only two hundred children affected by AT, the people at the AT Society know Graham and Carole well. So the genetic counsellor is going to contact us, and we might also talk to the professor there. The chances of us both being carriers is very small, so it's probably unrelated. But at least this way we'll be able to rule it out as a factor.

Then came the most difficult hour yet – meeting the funeral directors. Although Mum offered her support, we were brave and decided we needed to do this on our own. Now we have to design our son's funeral. It's unbelievable how many decisions have to be made. We've managed to decide on the time the services will take place and where Finley will be buried. But there's so much more. We need to get Finley there. While he can travel in the car with us, someone else will have to drive. We need to settle on who will carry his coffin into the church. And select the music and hymns.

I've been spending time trying to find the right music. I want Baz to choose something too, but need to find the best time to talk to him. He seems to have left this up to me. Mind you, he's decided he wants a Plymouth Argyle wreath! I suppose football was always going to come into it somewhere.

We have to choose a coffin. A coffin for our baby boy. I mean, how can a person choose that? I didn't even know people made coffins for babies. But the funeral directors gave us a brochure. It's for a company called Colourful Coffins. And we've chosen a lovely design. On it, a little boy is holding a teddy bear loosely in his hands as he floats away on a kite from a cliff into a deep blue sky. While it's sad, it carries real meaning for us. We imagine it's Finley flying his kite at the Seven Sisters.

We can order the coffin in a larger size, they inform us. That way we can put things inside it with Finley. I want to include a letter and a poem to Finley, but I don't know where I'll find the strength to write them. I'd like Baz to write something too. Still, I'm not sure he'll agree. I want to write a letter to God. To ask him to look after my little man. This is strange because I don't even know if I believe in God. Or the Universe. Or anything really.

Finley is supposed to come back from Bristol today, and should be at the hospital by now. The funeral directors will collect him as soon as they receive the coffin. He has been traumatised enough, they say. So they will move him just one more time. Let him be at peace.

I don't want to think about my baby being traumatised. Only of him as peaceful and sleeping. So the conversation makes me imagine all the awful things they are doing to him over in Bristol. I've had clinical training and know what it's like to dissect bodies. Now my mind has linked those memories to my own baby. It's horrific.

They tell us we can see Finley whenever we want. But I don't think I will. I am so anxious about what he'll look like after the post-mortem. I'm imagining all sorts. Maybe I'll call the labour ward tomorrow. I can ask them to visit Finley and describe him to me.

Now I'm starting to think I'd like to bring Finley home the night before the funeral. He'll see his bedroom. And we'll light our candle for him. But I can't make up my mind. I want us to spend time together as a family, but I'm afraid I won't be able to let him go. I don't know if I can walk away from him again.

A funeral is supposed to commemorate a life. To celebrate it. But how can you commemorate something that hasn't happened? Celebrate a life that hasn't been lived? What was it Carolyn said about me having an intuitive sense of Finley? Ah yes, she suggested I may have had an awareness of what he was like and the kind of personality he had. She's right. I know Finley. I know him really well. I have always known him.

When I had Reiki during my pregnancy, I connected with Finley very deeply. Finley is peaceful, happy, wise and clever. He has many great things ahead of him. And yet I don't know how I can express this at the funeral. So, while I do feel in a way that the funeral can be a celebration, I also know for certain that it can't be a happy one. I can't try and make it pleasant for others when I feel as unhappy as I do. At the very least, I hope we'll manage to get across a feeling of peace.

The appalling thing is that I feel as though I started preparing for this before it happened. I mean, how come I just know the right songs to use? I've gone for You Can Relax Now by Susan Mccullen. I sang it to Finley when he was inside me and could hear my voice. You can relax now...I am with you my sweet, sweet child...You thought we were separate. But now you hear my voice. It's beautiful. I would have sung him to sleep with it. It feels so natural to have the song play when we carry our baby into the church. So easy to imagine singing it to him while he sleeps in the coffin. I don't understand why. I just hope he can still hear my voice.

After the miscarriage, we couldn't even listen to the Foo Fighters' song Home. Yet now I hear it and straight away I see the photo slide-show that could accompany it at the funeral. Once I received a digital vision board from a friend: it had music, words and pictures attached. Now all I see is how easy it will be to use it to make a tribute to our baby boy. Why? How come when I went to a graveyard once, I found myself at the baby garden with all the teddy bears and small, colourful graves? Why did I feel so peaceful there? As if I was searching for something?

All these questions. I haven't any answers.

To Finley,

Hello sweetheart. I have started writing notes to you. I have so much I want to say. You have come back to be closer to us today, yet it still seems as if you are too far away. You should be back from the post-mortem, and I am so scared that you saw it, felt it, or that they have hurt you. I feel so guilty for putting your tiny little body through it, but we need to find out why this happened to you.

I hope that you like the bed we have chosen for you to go to sleep in. We will find you a fluffy warm outfit to wear in it. I love you so much and hope you can feel that love. Night night Angel. Come and visit me in your dreams.

Day 9

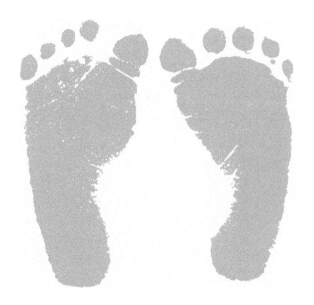

We went shopping in Bristol to buy Finley the outfit he will wear forever. The clothes we will bury him in. I wanted to get them in Mamas and Papas. It's an expensive shop and, when I was pregnant, we used to wander the aisles dreamily, never buying a thing. Still, we couldn't find anything we liked, so tried Mothercare. Walking around brought back all my memories of being pregnant when we had everything to look forward to. Now, all I see is expectant couples, parading their bumps with no idea how lucky they are.

Instead of opting for warm and fluffy, we've chosen something really smart. A tiny white shirt with a granddad collar, a pair of brown trousers and a grey waistcoat. The shirt has brown and grey stripes, so the whole outfit matches beautifully. It's just the kind of thing I imagine we'd have bought for Finley to wear at Baz's best friend Joanne's wedding next month. To complete the outfit, we found a pair of tiny, fluffy grey boots. Now Finley's feet won't get cold. By the time we left the shops, I'd found a small teddy bear and comforter blanket to go into Finley's coffin with him. Also a sweet card with a black-and-white photo of a baby on it. Beneath it the words Softly Sleeping Baby Boy.

Day 10

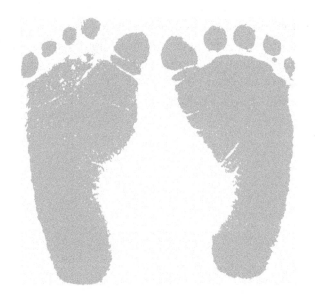

It's Dad's birthday and things are totally different to the way I'd imagined they would be. For a start, I didn't know what to write in the birthday card. I still wanted to sign Finley's name, just as we had that summer for Dad's Father's Day card. Of course, we hadn't known then that we were going to have a boy, so the card read from Mel, Baz and Flump. Nothing seems fair any more.

Old friends from our clubbing days, Darren and Hayley, Chloë, Mandy and Sam took it in shifts to visit this evening. Chloë gave us a great little photo frame. We all sat together looking through our photos and videos of Finley. At one point, Darren got up and left the room. It was all too hard on him. Darren and Hayley's three-month-old daughter Amber had had the umbilical cord wrapped around her neck during a difficult delivery. Despite the complications and her small six-pound birth weight, Amber survived.

It's tough trying to make sense of this. Amber was tiny and had the cord wrapped around her neck. Finley was three pounds heavier and there were no comparable problems. But he didn't stay with us. I wish Amber and Finley could both be here, playing together.

It strikes me as odd that, even though this has happened to us, we are not the only people who are affected by it. Everyone who knows us is moved. Chloë and Stu, whose baby girl Honey is around Amber's age, were very emotional. Sam and Mandy cried at the photos too. Maybe it's because they know our story. They've watched us from the time we first started trying to get pregnant, then as we suffered the miscarriage and hoped for a baby a second time.

Day 11

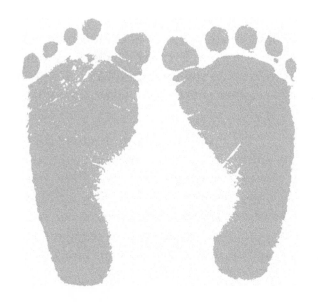

The people at Colourful Coffins have been in touch. The coffin should be with the funeral directors tomorrow. Apparently, the silver wreath holders we've ordered are too large to fit on Finley's tiny coffin. How could we have known? We barely know what's supposed to happen at a baby's funeral. I'm finding it extremely painful having to deal with such things. Things I never could have dreamt of having to do. I hope no one else ever has cause to imagine them either.

The funeral directors say they can design the funeral service sheets to match the picture on Finley's coffin. On the back, they're going to put the photograph of the three of us. Our little family. I'm pleased they're going to do that as I want everyone to see how beautiful our son was.

We gave Finley's little outfit to Debbie, the funeral director. She had washed his blanket for me because it had blood on it from the hospital which upset me terribly. I'd tried to wash the blood out myself when I was there, but there was no washing powder. When the coffin arrives, Debbie will call us so we can go and see our little boy at last. I want to see him desperately. I'm still worried about what he'll look like, but can't stand the thought of never being able to see him again. Still, I know the time will come all too soon. The very last time I ever see my baby. So I have decided for certain now that I want to bring Finley home the night before the funeral. I hope Baz is okay with it. He isn't really talking about what he wants. I just hope it's all okay.

We went back to the hospital to say thank you to the maternity staff and let them know when we're having the funeral. I managed to get hold of the names of the two other wonderful midwives (Pauline and Angela) so that we can send a card to them as well as Jill and Sandra. It's almost impossible to believe that nearly two weeks have passed since Finley was born. I really had to stop to think when the midwife asked me for the date he was born. I'd already said on Sunday before I realised it was actually one week ago last Sunday.

The midwife kindly suggested I may want to spend time in The Conway Suite. Since Baz didn't want to come this time, I went alone. Curiously, I couldn't find my own way there, despite the three days I'd been in the suite just less than a fortnight ago. I walked in and instantly felt very much at peace. Instantly reconnected with Finley. I could sense him in my arms, picture him in his cot and in the bath we gave him. Waves of tears washed down my face. It was an incredible experience; I hadn't expected it. It felt so valuable to me that I wonder whether we'll be able to go back another time. I just hadn't expected to feel such serenity in a place like that. Nothing like a hospital at all.

Later, Mum and I chose a second pair of matching shoes for Finley to wear. Mum feels guilty she isn't giving us something special to put into the coffin. So I showed her Baz's Plymouth Argyle teddy bear and the book that Beverley (his mum) and her partner Mick had sent. It's David Van Buren's I Love You As Big as the World. Inside, Beverley has written a really moving passage saying how much Finley was loved despite the short time he spent on earth and in her arms. Mum asked whether she might put the bear she'd given us at the hospital into the coffin. But I want to keep that because it's one of the few things we have saying Congratulations On Your Baby Boy. While I would never want this to happen to anyone I know, if it does, I'll be sure to send a card congratulating them on the birth of their baby. One of the best things you can do to support parents grieving a loss such as ours is acknowledge the baby as a person. No matter how short a time that baby was here.

Mum said she liked the announcement we'd put in the newspaper: Barry and Melanie Scott are proud to announce the birth of Finley John Scott, who sadly did not wake up. The details of the funeral followed. We kept hold of a copy and Mum's put the announcement into her photo album.

We went to the florist too, and while there I was struck by the sense that this is the way things are meant to be. Baz had been looking for a flower arrangement in the shape of a teddy bear wearing a Plymouth Argyle t-shirt but our local florist hadn't been able to help. However, this florist was far more positive and handed us a selection of brochures. As soon as I opened one, right there staring back at me was a flower teddy in Argyle strip, complete with hat and scarf! So we've ordered it and given the florist a badge to pin to the kit too.

I'd wanted to get an arrangement that spelt out Son, but the letters weren't right. The florist advised us against them anyway as they're so big they'd dwarf Finley's coffin. I saw a 3D stand-up bear that I liked too, but it turned out that would be too large as well. We could hardly have anticipated complications like these, let alone have been capable of dealing with them on our own. Luckily, the florist showed us a heart-shaped arrangement with Mum spelt out in pink flowers which I've chosen to have made up as Son in blue and white flowers with thistles (we had them in our wedding bouquet). I like it that Finley's funeral is close to the anniversary of our wedding. It makes him part of the family. Perhaps in future we'll turn the whole week into our own special family week.

We shed a few tears when writing the cards. Baz wrote Luv you always. Be good up there. No kicking the footballs at the pearly gates. What a comical image he's come up with! He clearly expects our little boy to be a hooligan! My note is quite different: To my darling little boy Finley John Scott. Here for such a short time, loved forever. Sleep well my angel. Love, Mummy. I must make sure I use Finley's name often, as it's still a struggle to say it out loud. It's almost as though it doesn't belong to him since it's so unfamiliar to me.

I've eaten twice today – a definite improvement. With so little appetite this far, I've already shrunk back to my pre-pregnancy weight and my tummy is almost gone. The midwife commented on it the other day. But I'm feeling angry at my body. I know I should be happy. I'm sure I would be happy if only I had my baby here with me. It's just that right now this feels like a kick in the teeth. As if Finley was never here.

The thing is, I actually feel really connected to Finley. My friend Tania even told me earlier that she's challenged by quite how physically connected I was to him. I'm sure we'll talk about it more later. I get the impression this is something really important. The connection seems absolutely natural, instinctive. After all, he grew inside my body.

This extra special connection with Finley is bringing me closer to other people in unexpected ways too. For instance, I've just started talking again with a friend I knew at school. I've discovered she's lost babies too. And it's as if we've never been apart. Both of us find we're especially close to our families right now. A good friend of mine who's also a highly regarded family therapist, has told me that Finley's purpose is to heal the past. I think he may be right. Out of the blue, I had a message from my ex-boyfriend. He said he was sorry to hear about Finley. For years I'd been frightened of this man, fearful that he'd find me and come and harm me. Now I no longer have that fear. All the negativity has vanished. As soon as he'd expressed his sympathies, I knew he couldn't possibly be holding onto his negative feelings towards me any more.

To Finley,

I have felt like I am with you today.

Day 12

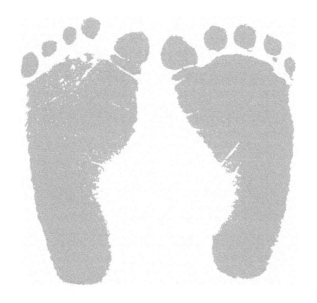

It's been a bad day. I've cried a lot, and when I start I can't stop. People make me cry when they talk to me because they always seem to be crying too.

I like Jade's idea of bringing a windmill to the funeral on Monday. I've not decided what else to put on Finley's grave yet. It's enough of a struggle choosing what he'll have with him in the coffin. I can only take one step at a time. Still, I do know that I want to write a letter for the coffin. I need to write a letter to my baby. I want to tell him about all the things I dreamt we would share. All the things he could do and have. To tell him how amazing he would have been.

If only I had a solid belief system to reassure me that Finley will be back with us again one day. Faith that all those wishes could come true. That my hopes could be fulfilled. I'd love to believe that. Or that each choice we make produces a different life-strand so that at any given moment there are other worlds out there where we're all, in fact, still together. But I don't. I don't believe it. Everyone else seems to have a fair idea what I could or should believe in right now. But I can't subscribe to any of it. It all seems far closer to delusion than truth. Just stuff I need to believe because I'm suffering so much.

It's true there are times I believe Finley's soul will be back on earth again. Times I believe that in his short visit with us, he did the job he needed to do this time round. I certainly feel I've met him before, and know for sure that he was a peaceful, wise, old soul. I'm comforted by the thought that others will be blessed to meet him too. Things happen for a reason, I know it. So many good things have already come out of the last two weeks. But right now, these tentative beliefs of mine are pretty much shattered. Nothing changes my wish that things could be different. I simply can't believe that Finley will come back to us. It's just not true and that's devastating.

Baz told me he doesn't want to write a letter to Finley. He's not ready to say goodbye. He'll find his own way when the time is right. I know how important this is. Perhaps we'll walk up to the Seven Sisters together; it's always helped us to go there at difficult times.

Incredibly, I made it out for a coffee with friends. I was very quiet, and knew it, but they did a great job of keeping the conversation going. We drove back past the cemetery where Finley will be buried on Monday. Some of the managers from work will be there. My colleagues have sent me flowers. Our five bookshelves plus mantelpiece are now littered with cards. I'm going to need to hang some up with string. I'm comforted that people are thinking of us. But I'm overwhelmed by just how many.

I agreed to talk to Baz's cousin Nina tonight. I didn't want to talk to her: I knew she'd be nice. It's a struggle when people are so nice all the time. It's not that they're usually unpleasant of course. It's just that, now, it's a different sort of kindness and I find it hard to handle. Everyone keeps saying how brave we are. It doesn't feel like they're talking about us at all. This isn't bravery. It's not even coping.

I spent time online, reading websites full of poems and other people's stories of grief and loss. I can't decide yet whether it's a form of self-punishment or if it's helping me cope. That said, I do wonder what on earth it can be that's getting me through the days. I can barely sleep or eat. I hardly drink a drop of water. It must be adrenalin, and pretty soon I'm going to fall asleep for a long, long time.

We didn't sleep last night either. Just lay holding each other for a long time. I love touching Baz, cuddling him. Our relationship is everything. Wow, I can't see how I can even consider having sex at a time like this. It feels wrong. Like dishonouring our baby's memory. We only lost him a couple of weeks ago.

As I say this, I can feel my hormones going crazy. They're buzzing all over the place. In so many ways right now, I feel deeply alive. More so than ever before. Plus I don't even give my body image a second thought any more. I feel good. And I can't think of a better way to kick death in the teeth.

To Finley,

Our time together is running out. It's now just two full days until Monday. And I know these will be days when I'll be required to do lots of things that will take my attention away from you. I hope we can come to see you tomorrow.

We have been brave enough to say that we want you to come home on Sunday. I want to show you your room, your toys and your books. I know that I want to hold you all through the night, to hold you for as long as I can. You fit the space between my arms perfectly.

The candle we've ordered with your sweet photo will arrive tomorrow and we will light it for you on Sunday. Then it will be specially protected and can go on your grave if we want. The flame signifies your light that will always be with us.

It's funny, but I have this urge to rush round tomorrow tidying up for when you come home! And you know how unusual that is for me.

Day 13

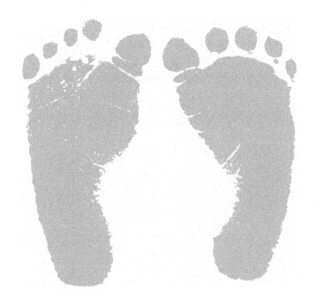

Another very hard day for me after staying up late drinking vodka with Baz. I got up to find three-quarters of the bottle gone (oops!), and a hubby with a hangover. He actually gave me a lecture about drinking too much! I think he's forgotten I haven't had a single drink in nine months.

Finley is now in the Chapel of Rest. I was anxious about going to see him there, but knew I needed to. I'm thankful I did. In fact, I'm keeping in mind the saying that you never regret what you have done, but what you haven't. It's helping me find the courage to do everything I need to do right now, however demanding. If I don't do these things now, neither of us will have the chance again. I'm acutely aware of this fact. I needed to see Finley in his coffin today, because I need to know he's dead. At times this week it's been as though he's not dead at all. And, although I sometimes feel that he was never here, mostly the sensation is one of him being present but not with me. It's heartbreaking.

It was different when we were in hospital. Those three days were like time out from the world. Just Finley, Baz and me. Finley was with me, sleeping. At least that's how it felt. It was a precious time. At night, it was so easy to believe he was going to wake up very soon. There I was, cuddling my beautiful baby. All alone with him in that peaceful little place. Sometimes people visited, permeating our little bubble for a moment. But mostly, it was just us.

I can remember it; I need to remember it. To piece it all together. The hazy memories of the first day when I was on morphine and sleeping. Holding Finley when someone passed him to me. Phoning a couple of friends; worrying them. Feeling numb. Baz staying the night on a pull-out mattress on the floor. The two of us taking turns to cuddle Finley. Realising after the initial shock that I wanted to hold my baby and not let him go. Never letting him lie alone in his cot so long as we were awake. Handing him to Baz while I hobbled to the toilet. Wrapping him tightly in his fluffy blanket and putting him in his cot as he held onto his teddy bear. Waking throughout the night to ask the midwives to help me sit up or lie down, go to the toilet or take more pain killers. Baz deciding to go home the following night.

That last night in hospital was the most precious. I remember every second. At eight thirty, Jill popped in to say goodnight. She would let Angela know our wishes for the following day, so that she could support us as we prepared to leave. Then Jill offered to take some photos of us. They're in black and white and softly lit. Jill directed me, suggesting I hold Finley's hand and stroke his face. She also said I might want to kiss him and I did. My first time. I cherish that photo now. All the photos are deeply moving. More so than any I've ever seen. Each one makes me sob now, seeing Finley all snuggled up to me, the tears streaming down my face.

I didn't let Finley go all night long. I couldn't take my eyes off him. If I had to get out of bed, I would place him in his cot really carefully, then pick him up again immediately as I got back in. I knew he was dead, but I just had to hold him. I had no choice – it was the right thing to do. The only thing to do. Finley's shape fitted into the crook of my arm perfectly. Even now at night I can feel the weight of him there. I remember thinking how lucky I was to be able to sleep with my baby in bed with me. Parents are normally advised against it. So I lay in bed, nursing my baby in my arms, making sure he was wrapped up in his blanket. Sometimes, when I moved him, his nose would bleed and I would wipe it with a wet wipe. The bleeding was a sign that Finley's body was starting to break down, but for me it was a chance to care for my baby.

When I talk about this, I worry. I worry what people will think of a mother holding her dead baby for three days straight. I worry what they'll think about me wiping away the blood from his nose with a baby wipe. I worry that people might think it's wrong. Or just too tragic. Like one of those straight-to-TV movies based on a true story. But I won't ever forget those three days. They helped me acknowledge just how perfect my son was. I had an instinctive need to hold him and look after him and I just had to allow myself to do it. I vaguely remember someone asking if I wanted him put in the morgue. I couldn't even consider it. Part of me, deep down, knew our time was limited. And I wanted every second of it.

Seeing Finley in the chapel has been a different kind of experience. Things have changed. Finley has changed. He looks different. Still as peaceful as he did in the hospital. But now he is very definitely dead. I could see it today very clearly for the first time. He was cold, his skin a different colour. My son is dead but I am still deeply connected with him. I am still his mother. I love my son as any mother would. The feelings don't just stop because he is dead. When I look at Finley, all tucked up with his teddy bears in the coffin, he looks cute. His little outfit looks gorgeous. He was wearing the blue hospital hat, so I started wondering if the one we bought didn't fit or if the blue one wouldn't come off. I couldn't help worrying about his feet being cold either, since even though he was wearing the fluffy boots, he didn't have any socks on. Typical mother. I can almost hear Finley telling me to stop fussing Mum!

The coffin is more lovely than we'd imagined. It's shiny and very hard, and makes me feel Finley's going to be safe. We've taken photos of Finley in it. The Green Army teddy bear is by his head, he's holding a little blue bear in one hand, and the blanket in his other. Just like any other baby holding onto his toys when he goes to sleep. Now he's got a little elephant comforter from Mum, and a small journey bear from the people at Colourful Coffins. They've attached a card saying I was sent to be with you. Beverley's book won't fit into the coffin, so we're going to put it on the top. I want to remember every little detail. Whether it seems weird to anyone else or not.

We spoke to Martin, the vicar, about the funeral preparations. I can barely comprehend that almost three years ago we were here planning our wedding. Sitting on the same sofa, stroking the same dog. Martin was fantastic. He listened to us; he understood what we wanted. He'll select the readings, and will include the verse that was in the chaplain's card (the one that goes when you were in the womb I knew you). It's true, when he was in my womb, I knew Finley. It was the only time we shared. The verse is addressed to a Christian God, but it feels like it's me, like it's coming from me.

We'll sing Make Me a Channel of your Peace. It feels as though I always knew we would, that somehow I was ready for this. We'd sung the same hymn at our wedding, and at Nana Brooks' funeral. I love the words, although I'm sure they'll feel forever altered on Monday. We'll light a candle at the church and Martin will give Finley his name. It's not a christening as such, but a small naming ceremony in a church nevertheless. And this really matters to me. It feels vital. When he's called by his name – officially – it's real. Finley really does exist.

Martin will talk about the baby we lost last year too. I'd like to discuss naming our first baby with Baz. Even if it's something silly like Poppet. We didn't think about it at the time; there wasn't long enough. But I'd definitely like Martin to refer to her by name during the service. Just one thought of Mother's Day next year and I'm weeping uncontrollably. I'll know I should have been getting a card from my new baby when all I'll have is an empty space in my arms where he should've been.

Martin talked about sleep, asking is it helpful, or not, to consider death a kind of sleep? He believes Finley will wake up, but that we won't be there to see it. I'm glad he has this faith, and hope it helps me find my own, whatever form it takes. Right now, it all confuses me. The words don't make sense. People refer to stillborn babies as babies born sleeping. It's totally unclear. Does the baby ever wake up? Or does his soul awaken while his body stays sleeping? Still, I guess I'm going to have a lot of time, a lot of sleepless nights, to think about all this stuff.

To Finley,

Monday is getting closer. I don't want to let you go. I am so silly. I'm still wearing my hospital band because I don't want to cut that tie to you. We saw your body today, and you look so peaceful. I wonder where you are, because I know you're not there in that body any more. It's just the shell that held you for a blessed forty-one weeks and five days.

If we let you go, will you be able to come back and visit us? We've been so convinced that there's a ghost of a little girl in our house. She visits us occasionally — will you come back and play with her?

I hope you are happy, my little one, and that I will feel your wonderful soul/spirit/essence near me. I know I will think of you when the wind blows, when the sun's rays cut through the clouds, or a butterfly flutters across my path.

My heart is full to bursting with my love for you. I never knew it was possible to love someone this much. I hope you will still feel that love (the vicar says you will), and that you are lifted away from us when you are ready on a rainbow of our love. A love that will never end. A love that's a rainbow because it includes both sunshine and rain (good times and bad, darkness and light, happiness and sadness). We need this mix, because out of it comes balance. And in the balance is beauty.

At this moment I am absolutely connected with you. I don't understand this mentally. I just feel it. When I start to think it hurts in my stomach and I can't feel you. I don't want to stop writing — I have so much to say to you. I feel I've got to say it all before Monday even though I know I'll continue talking to you as long as I have breath to speak, or thoughts to write down. How can you have been here for such a short time and have had such a huge impact? So many things have happened since last week. You should be here so we can thank you. I love you little one.

Day 14

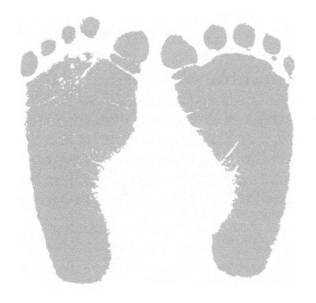

My first two visitors today – Bianca, then Barb, the midwife – were happy to talk about the funeral and bringing Finley home. Barb reckons we're an inspiration. We're being so strong, she says. I know that's what everyone thinks, but I still don't feel brave or strong. I feel as if I'm in pieces. Barely surviving. All I'm doing is what needs to be done, whatever I can do while we still have the time. It's basic self-preservation. I don't want to have any regrets.

I pottered around vacuuming and tidying Finley's room, just like any other mum really. At two-thirty, Peter the funeral director arrived. He came in alone to take us through the order of service. It's just right. While there's nothing to stop us, he advised us not to take Finley out of the coffin. By now, Finley really has been messed about with quite enough and should be left to be at peace. It was a relief to hear Peter say this, because if I were to hold Finley again, I know I wouldn't ever want to let him go.

Finally Peter brought Finley into the house. Home at last. He carried Finley upstairs, placing the coffin into the cot. Ah yes, he said, that feels like the right place. And it does. Little Finley has come home to be with us, his family, for the last time. I wept, of course I did. Lighting Finley's candle, listening to all the songs that'll be played tomorrow when we say our final goodbyes – I cried my heart out. The lyrics are breathtaking. They say it all.

Now Finley has five teddy bears in his coffin with him. I've just unwrapped another from Jade – it's a Tigger. She'll have got Finley a Tigger because he was always bouncing around inside me when I was pregnant. I didn't unwrap it until now because I wanted to wait until Finley was here with me before I opened his presents. They're his presents after all. I'm crushed that all I can do is describe them to him; crushed that he'll never get to play with them. Jade has also given Finley two tokens – one for a hug and one for a kiss. So I've put one in his tiny hand.

As I watch him, can't take my eyes from him, Finley still looks asleep. Still peaceful. Just as he did in the chapel. But he is empty now. In the hospital, I felt like Finley was still with his body. But now his body is dead, and Finley is gone. You can see it – I need to see it. First in the Chapel of Rest. Now here, in his own cot. Finley is cold, and the skin around his mouth has darkened. But his hands are perfect. They're a more normal colour now, apart from the nails which are dark purple, very long and pointed. Without these few signs, it'd be all too easy to believe Finley is still here. All the same, I've been holding his hand, telling him what's going to happen tomorrow. Reading him his card from Beverley's best friend Joyce. Talking about his presents. Now that his body is here with me, I can acknowledge that Finley is dead. Yet at the same time, I can also experience the very live connection I have with him even now.

What's amazing is how much Finley being here is helping other people with their grief too. Beverley and Mick spent a while alone with him tonight. Then, at seven, we all went into his room, listened to the songs, and each lit a candle. A real taste of what it'll be like tomorrow with a whole room of people crying. Finley is a much-loved baby.

When our old friend Jodie and her husband Craig visited, Jodie and I chatted about Billy, her nephew, who died last year. Jodie came up to Finley's room with me. Seeing Finley and saying goodbye to him really comforted her. We stood for a long time next to Finley's cot, holding each other.

I've been trying to write my letter to Finley all day long. I just can't get going with it. I want to sleep in the bed in Finley's room so he's not on his own. I don't think Baz wants to join me.

> To Finley,
>
> You are home with us and that is enough.

Day 15

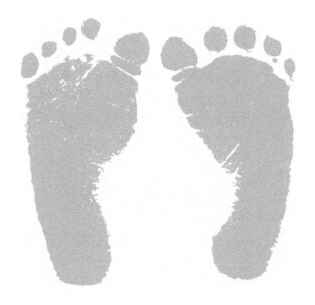

Last night was really something special. Finley was at last resting in his cot, tucked into his cosy coffin filled with teddies. Serene and at peace. Eventually, I found the words I needed to write him a letter. The candle stayed lit for him for a long, long time.

Baz had pulled out the bed so I could stay in the room. I curled up in bed with Finley's fluffy blanket. I couldn't sleep, but felt tranquil as I sang to him, and shared my thoughts with him. While I was looking at Finley's coffin, I felt his presence behind me. Just to the left where his candle stood. In the light. It was the same spot I used to sense Finley in during Reiki. Exactly the same place the psychic had seen a spirit. I've decided to go and visit her again.

Finley's room was warm and hush, filled with the flickering candlelight. I put my hospital bracelet into his hand together with the hug token. I'd been wearing the band since I left hospital, feeling it connected me to him, showing that I'm his mum. It's right that he carries it with him now. Into Finley's tiny, perfect hand, I put the rose quartz crystal heart Tania and Carolyn had given me. I'd been wearing it since hospital too. I've held it just as I've held Finley, and meditated on it. In fact, I've been wearing rose quartz in some form since I first knew I wanted to be a mum. It symbolises love.

Before going to bed, we left a message on our event wall on Facebook:

The candle is lit in your bedroom, watching over you as you sleep in your bed. Know that we will light your candle often and think of you. Each time we see the flame dance, we will know it is your breath that makes it so. We will be comforted by the fact that whether the light is bright or dim, it never has to go out.

I imagine you on your own little rainbow tomorrow, watching us. A rainbow cannot exist without sunshine and rain. It is the beauty that lies in the balance between the two. Just like the rainbow, you, Finley, are the beauty that arises when sadness and joy come together.

We love you forever Finley.

But that was last night. I've said nothing yet about today. About what's happened. I'm avoiding it. Because today we watched as our baby boy was buried. Today our lives changed forever. Today what passes for normality has been forever altered. I don't know if things are better or worse now. Or if everything is just unknown.

First thing, Peter arrived along with three cars. I put the sleeping baby card into Finley's coffin. Inside, I'd written To whom it may concern. Please look after Finley John for us. He is coming to be an angel, to be the change we wish to see in the world. He will show people how to love. Until we can look after him again. Love from Finley's Mummy and Daddy. Peter screwed down the lid.

The flowers had been laid out in the back of the car. Baz's Plymouth Argyle teddy bear was fantastic. Next to it was the heart I'd chosen spelling out Son in beautiful purple flowers. We rode in the back seat, holding hands over Finley's coffin.

We were met at the church by a whole crowd of people. Everyone hugged us. My strong, brave Baz decided to carry the coffin into the church. It broke my heart to witness such courage. You Can Relax Now was playing over the loudspeakers as we walked in. I was thankful we didn't have to listen to it all. So, Finley's coffin stood at the front of the church on a stool, surrounded by all the flowers and two lit candles. His book from Nana was placed next to him, and a Plymouth Argyle sticker from his uncle stuck to the coffin.

We were lucky to have the wonderful Martin as our vicar. He happily made last minute changes to include a reading of the letter I'd written Finley. Despite the crowd, it felt as if it was just me, Baz and Finley in the church. No one else mattered. I couldn't let go of Baz and couldn't take my eyes off Finley. Then, just as Home by the Foo Fighters came over the speakers, Baz began to cry. At that, I simply couldn't stop myself, and I wept and wept infinite tears. I'm glad Baz cried. He's been so strong for me that I was worried he's been bottling everything up inside.

The vicar read Do Not Cry For Me My Parents, the poem my friend Raphael had written especially for Baz and me:

Do not cry for me my parents,

For I am not lost, nor alone;

Do not cry for me my father,

For I am always here

Your rock and your stone.

Do not grieve for me my mother,

For I am always at your side.

I live inside of you both,

and my soul eternal glides,

amongst the stars, and moonlit nights

and in the shards of light.

Look out upon the heavens

For you will see me soaring there;

It was not my time dear mother,

yet you should not despair.

For I will come when I am ready,

and the time is right for me.

I live inside you both,

for now my soul is free.

So do not grieve for me Mother,

do not hang your heart in Woe,

For now I travel amongst the stars,

and Heaven is my home.

© Raphael. Monday, August 10th 2009

Next, my friend Fraser read out the letter I'd written to Finley.

To my darling Finley,

Thank you for coming to be with us. You have already made such a big impact on our lives with your short one. I don't think there has ever been another little person who is loved so much. Your daddy and me love you so very much – the book your Nana gave you says it all. We love you as big as the sky.

I know that when you ride your rainbow you will be joining your sister. You make sure you go and play with the horses at the Seven Sisters. We will go there; it's so high we will know you are there with us.

We will think of you when we see a rainbow – the beauty in the balance of sunshine and rain – or when we see a candlelight flicker, the rays of sunshine through the clouds, or a butterfly.

They say if a butterfly flaps its wings in Australia, a wind blows here – that's just like you. You never got a chance to flap your wings, but you sure made a change in the world. The world shines for me now; it is full of flickering candles for you, and so much love.

I want to thank you for coming to me. I loved being pregnant with you. I know you and all you would have been – all you will still be wherever you are. You are wisdom, peace happiness, joy and love. You are cheeky, mischievous and loveable. You are destined for wonderful things, amazing achievements, and a long, long future teaching others to love without conditions – without regrets. Just as you have taught me and your daddy. We love you.

Without condition; without regret.

It was a breathtaking moment. Mum asked for a copy of the letter. She was stunned I'd been able to write it. How had I found the words? Later, Debbie made copies. So now there's one letter in the ground with Finley, one in his memory box, and one stays with Mum.

I remember Mick reading out a poem he and Beverley had found. Then Martin speaking about love. Especially the love we've received from friends. He mentioned Facebook – that got a laugh. I mean, you don't expect a vicar at a funeral to start talking about

Facebook do you! As we'd agreed, Martin included Finley's sister in his sermon. It felt good and right that he should speak of them together. I recall him mentioning our wedding too. It was three years ago we'd said our vows in that same church. To conclude the service, we all sang Make me a Channel of your Peace. Falteringly.

Martin led our friends out, leaving family alone in the church. He was great. He played Faith Hill's There You'll Be first of all. In my dreams, I'll always see you soar above the sky. Singing the words to Finley gave me a deep sense of peace. Next came Barbra Streisand's If I Could, as Baz and I held onto each other in front of the coffin. If I could, I would try to shield your innocence from time, but the part of life I gave you isn't mine... I've watched you grow, so I could let you go. We gathered ourselves up and walked out.

Everyone wept. The songs were just too much, too moving. Even Debbie couldn't stop herself, despite having promised her husband she'd stay focused. Dad lost it too, and sobbed as the last song played. I felt guilty about it. I wanted people to feel better. Not so sad.

Still, there was a moment of normality and some laughter afterwards at the wake. The burial itself was over really quickly. Baz and his brother Ed lowered the coffin into the ground. I could never have done it. Finley's book, blanket and my letter went with him into his grave. We released three balloons (a last minute decision). Two baby-boy balloons and a heart-shaped one. They struggled to lift off since I'd tied all three together. Then one freed itself and started floating off alone before the others joined it. We laughed, saying that it was like Finley wanting to go his own way.

Now Finley lies under a hawthorn tree (I think it's a hawthorn anyway). There'll be blossoms in spring.

With all our friends back at the house, things felt almost normal. For a moment at least. Then I heard a baby crying in Finley's room. For the tiniest of seconds, I thought it was Finley and I started towards the room to settle him. Reality came crashing in when I realised it wasn't him. That I'd never get the chance to calm him when he cried. It was my friend Tamsin's five week old daughter Betsy. We'd suggested Tamsin could use the room for Betsy if she needed it. That room should have a baby in it.

As people started leaving, I was overcome and started crying again. Baz picked up little Betsy and gave her a cuddle. It broke my heart to see it. He should have a baby in his arms. His own baby. Finley. Life might well go back to its everyday routines for everyone else. But not for us. Other people might get up in the morning and trundle off to work. Not us. We'll be getting up to an empty house that should be filled with the sounds of a new baby. We'll be staring at empty arms when they should be full of hugs.

Curiously, despite feeling sick to my stomach most of the day and crying heaps, there have been moments I've felt profoundly still and serene. Moments when I stop thinking altogether. I want to be able to stop thinking more. Because when I think, I get agitated and frightened.

To Finley,

I hope you stayed with us today, and smiled as we let the balloons go at your grave.

I hope you are warm enough, and that you are not frightened. I hope your fluffy boots keep your feet warm, and I am sorry I did not find any socks. I should have asked someone to get some.

I hope you have someone with you as you start your next stage, and that you can come to visit us soon, and often.

We love you so very, very much. That love is timeless and spans any distance.

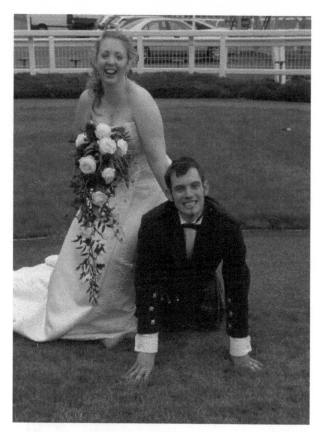

August 2006. Baz and I horsing around in the winners' circle at our wedding reception.

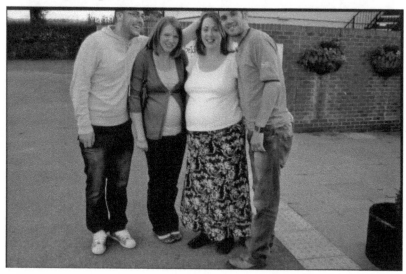

Pregnant together. With my brother and his girlfriend.

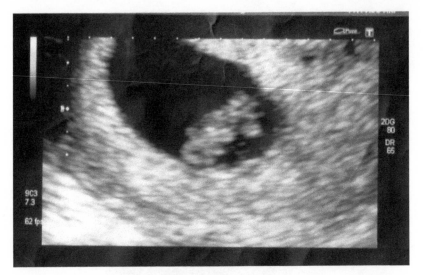

Our little seahorse (8 week scan).

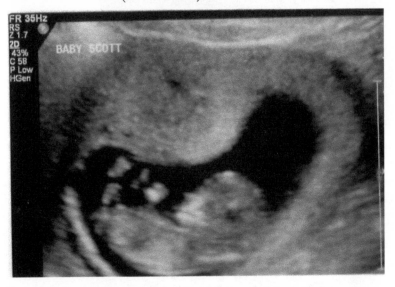

Lying back with his hand behind his head (12 weeks).

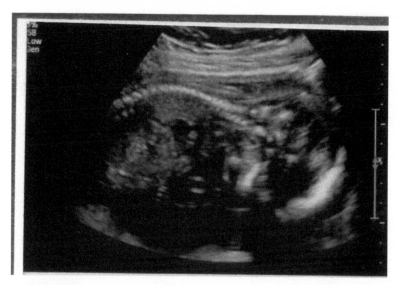

Keeping it secret: we waited until the birth to find out if we had a boy or girl (20 weeks).

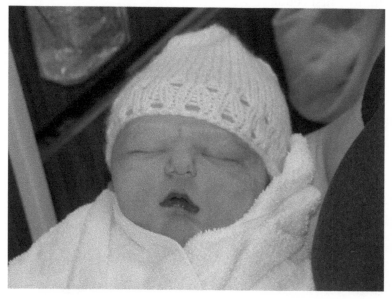

Day 1. Finley John Scott sleeping peacefully in Nana's arms.

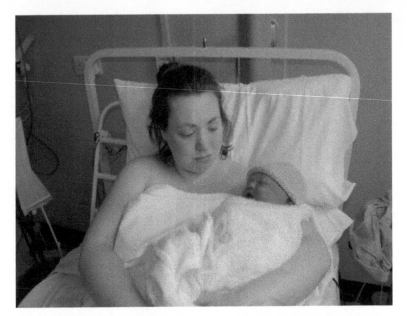

Mummy's first cuddle.

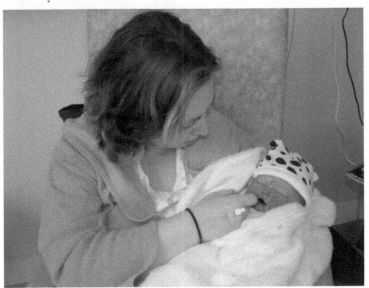

Day 2. Getting to know my son.

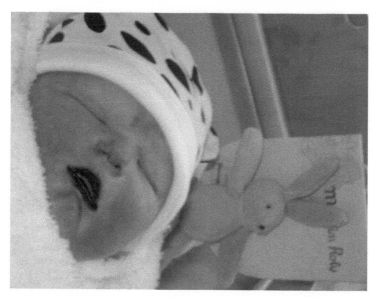

Day 3. Finley's first cuddly toy.

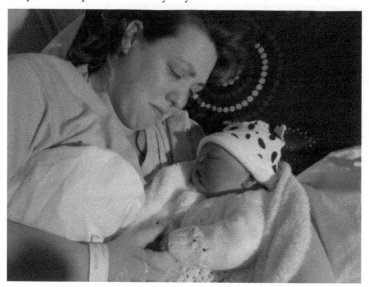

Holding Finley's hand.

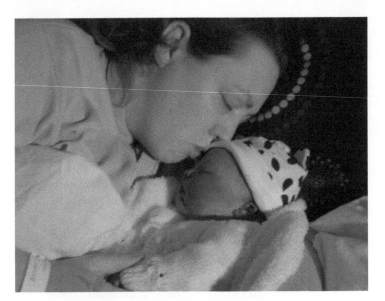

A kiss goodnight.

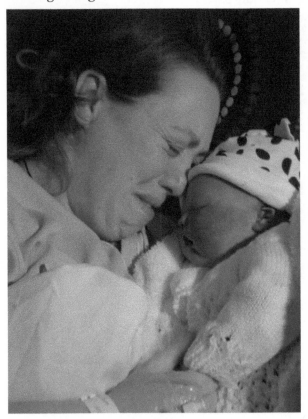

Knowing this can't last forever.

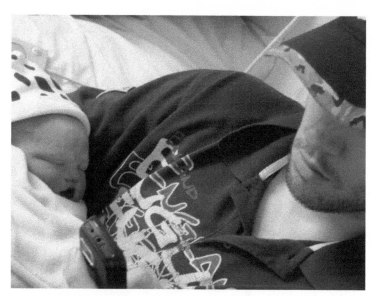

Day 4. Daddy's goodbye.

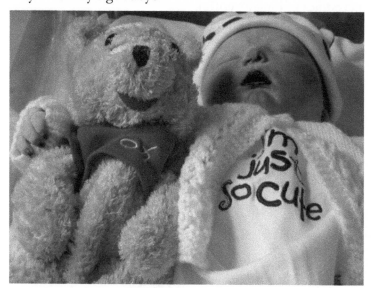

With Winnie-the-Pooh.

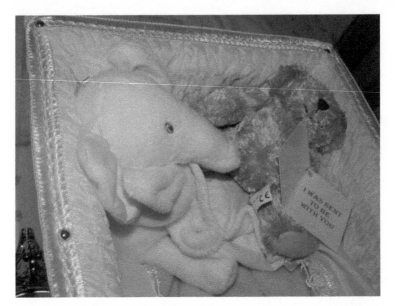

Day 14. Teddies in Finley's coffin.

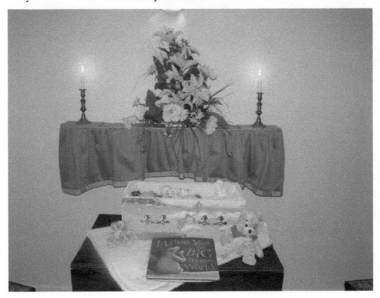

At the Chapel of Rest.

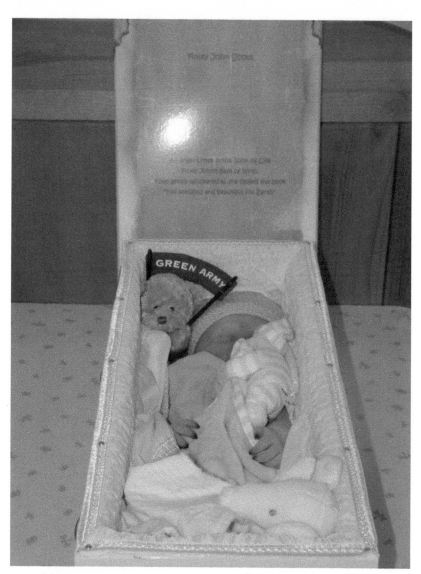

Day 15. Home at last.

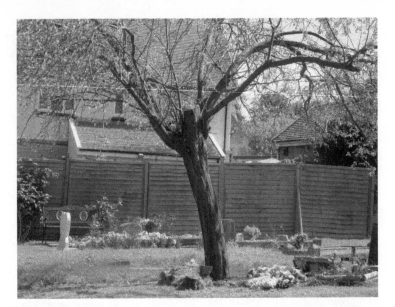

Day 19. Finley's final resting place under the hawthorn tree.

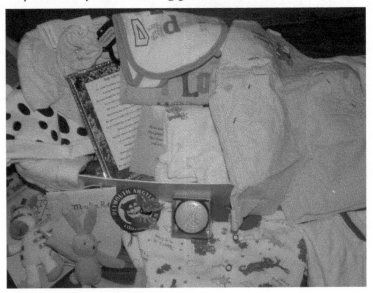

Memories are all we have left.

Day 16

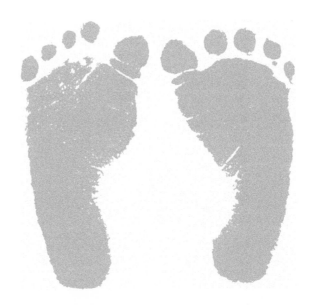

There's not much to write. It's nine-thirty at night and I've just woken up on the sofa. I haven't seen much of the day. I think I got up at lunchtime, ate half a bowl of Coco Pops and fell asleep again. We did go to see Baz's doctor though: we got Baz signed off for two weeks. Amazing that he'd be expected to go back to work tomorrow if we hadn't. We only buried our little boy yesterday. How could Baz possibly work? I can't see how he'll be able to go back even after another two weeks. It's hard enough to get through the most basic of functions like shopping. Seeing life going on for everyone else. While our life has stopped. The life we had imagined for ourselves has come to an end. People have left messages for us on Facebook. They're still thinking of us. They know it's not over. That helps.

It's our wedding anniversary tomorrow. We haven't had a chance to get each other cards, although we've received a few from others. I think we should postpone the anniversary and celebrate in a few weeks' time.

To Finley,

I have not been to see you today. It's too soon. I thought of you a lot last night. Silly Mummy is worried about you being on your own in the dark, or having cold feet, or being squashed with all the teddy bears! I can just imagine you shaking your head at me, saying Oh, Mum, you're so embarrassing. Daddy says he will visit you every weekend to read you the Plymouth Argyll football results – lucky you. I hope you like football.

Day 17

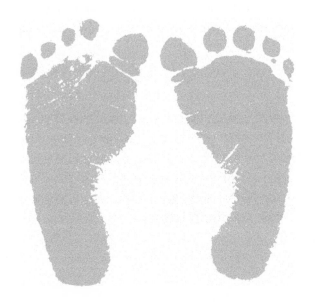

It should have been a beautiful day. Our third wedding anniversary. We should have been celebrating. We should have been sharing this anniversary with our sweet little baby boy Finley. He should have been two-and-a-half weeks old. We should have been exhausted because he'd kept us up all night demanding to be fed, or to get his nappy changed. We should have been going out for a meal in our favourite pub in the country with Finley asleep in his carry-cot. We should have been ravenous, wolfing down a scrummy three course meal. Things should have been the way we'd hoped and dreamed. But they're not.

We shouldn't have been exhausted, shaking and dizzy from not having eaten. We shouldn't have been this unhappy. We shouldn't have been trying to shop in Morrisons, despite feeling weak from lack of food. Suffering so badly every time we caught sight of a baby. You know, I feel an actual physical blow every baby I see. My stomach literally twists itself into knots – the true meaning of the word gut-wrenching. It's not surprising neither of us can find an appetite. We got a takeaway in the end, but left most of it on our plates.

Despite all this, somehow, I'm feeling less tearful, less detached, than I did yesterday. We've received presents from both our mums, and cards from friends too. Both mums had the same idea and got us a leather photo frame. From the same shop no less. The traditional theme for a third wedding anniversary is leather. Mum and I had a giggle earlier when she hinted that we might be making a trip to a rather 'special' shop. Baz just raised his eyebrows. What a relief my mate Sam hadn't known this is our leather anniversary. I can just picture her making references to horse whips, or Baz dressed in leather. I wouldn't put it past him either. I mean, this is the man who wore a donkey thong under his kilt at the wedding. The guy has no shame.

We'll need to decide where to hang the frames. We have so many photos to choose from. All of them photos of our baby, Finley. Dead and gone when he should be here with us.

We went to Finley's grave to take photos of the funeral flowers before they die. It's odd, I don't know if we're visiting his grave or if it's Finley himself we're going to see. The flowers are just the right size to cover the whole grave. There's no gravestone or anything with Finley's name on it yet. Just two windmills to mark my baby's grave. Baz and I checked out the graves nearby. It's pretty depressing, all those fresh flowers and many of the deaths so recent. Next to Finley are twin boys with just the one date on the gravestone - they must both have died the day they were born. Just along the row, there's a stone dated 1957. This stone looks new and the flowers are fresh. So there's still someone thinking of that poor baby more than fifty years on. It's daunting thinking that we'll still be visiting Finley and bringing him flowers fifty years from now. But we can't forget him. He's our baby and he lives on in our hearts.

Acknowledging this, a fearful thought that's been troubling me seems magically to have dissolved. I've been worrying what will happen if we move house? We dream of a beautiful country home with land so we can have animals for our children to look after, trees for them to climb. Now I realise we won't be leaving Finley behind when we move away. Finley's not in the body we buried here but will be with us wherever we are. If we want, we can devote a special place to him. Somewhere we can go to be close to him. We could buy another stone, just the same as his gravestone. Buy a plot for it in another cemetery. Or keep it on our woodland acreage, under its very own hawthorn tree.

So, instead of celebrating our anniversary, we went to the cemetery to visit our son and then to collect a catalogue from the place that makes gravestones. They were pleasant people, and the stones seemed fine. But we're not ready to choose. The prices are shocking, and Baz is devastated. He said that as Finley's dad he should be giving his boy the best. But there's no way he can afford a thousand pounds for a teddy bear gravestone with surround. I know that in some religions, a stone-setting ceremony is held a year after a death and the gravestone not laid until then. So I mentioned it to Baz. He still wants to have Finley's name there as soon as possible. Perhaps we can find a way to mark the grave while we save up for the perfect headstone. We want something special that we've chosen ourselves to mark Finley's last resting place. Not the cheapest stone we can find.

Then, a series of phone calls. Fraser called to see how we were. I thanked him for reading my letter to Finley at the funeral. I think

Fraser and Baz might become good friends. Fraser's offered to take Baz to watch some decent football. I'm sure Baz would love it. I can seriously imagine him showing Fraser how to party too.

I must've been chatting for almost three hours to my friend Alex, from London. We needed to catch up. She's been out of the country for, what, all of a week! She spoke frankly, and it was a relief at last to hear someone say you know what? this is awful; this is horrible. Mind you, I wouldn't want too many people saying it to me too often. Because it really is, you know. Horrendous. The worst possible experience. Finley should be here with us and he's not. It makes me uncomfortable just to say it. I can't help feeling superstitious now that I have said it; nervous that something even worse could happen. Worrying that I might have asked for it, just as I seem to have done when I've said similar things in the past.

The genetic counsellor from the AT Society rang and offered some reassurance. She says the society can test to see if Baz and Leonie carry the same genetic spelling mistake, but they can't test me since I'm not related to either Carole or Graham. Apparently, the chances of Finley having had AT are so, so tiny that it's unlikely the post-mortem will even check for it. She'd calculated all the genetic probabilities, far too complex for me to include here. Suffice to say there's less than a one percent chance that Finley had AT. Baz and I would both have to be carriers for him to have contracted it. It's also unknown for a child to die at birth from AT related complications. AT shows later, when the child starts walking. In fact, there's a two to three percent likelihood that any foetus is suffering from a genetic condition in the general population as a whole. So it's more likely that a baby of ours would have another genetic condition anyway.

None of this changes a thing. We're not interested in knowing whether or not Baz is a carrier. We'd never terminate a pregnancy by choice. It'd be like saying that Leonie's life is somehow not worth living. That kids like her and her brother Max (who has Down Syndrome) don't deserve a chance. That couldn't be further from the truth. Those kids are absolutely fantastic. They are deeply loved and very loving. Leonie's starting art college later this year, she's had a poem published in a book, and sends us cards and drawings all the time. We're close to her and had wanted her to be

Finley's godmother. She was so excited about the pregnancy and loves babies, even though she may never be able to have her own. More than anyone she deserved to get to know and spoil Finley. Honestly, people with genetic conditions may have a shorter life than those without them, but that doesn't mean it's a life any less worthwhile.

Still, I'm finding all this a little hard to digest. During my pregnancy, I used the affirmation I have a healthy baby. Now I'm anxious there was something wrong with Finley and that, because of my affirmation, he thought I didn't want him. That he left because we'd rejected him. A horrifying thought. Perhaps I just think about things too much. Way too much.

To Finley,

I have looked at the photos of you and me cuddling in the hospital today. I am so happy to have held you; to have known you. You and I look so much alike – especially our noses. You're so lucky you have my nose and not your dad's.

I wish I knew what colour eyes you have; I did wonder if I could lift your eyelids to have a look at them. I think that because you have blonde hair you would have had my blue eyes. You definitely would have been Mummy's little boy. You are Mummy's little boy.

Day 18

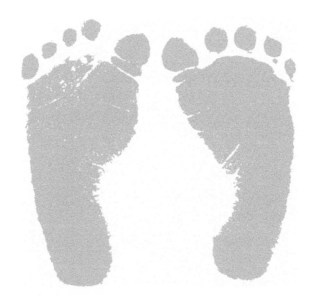

I say to my friend on Facebook, I'm having a hard day today. I can't eat, I feel sick and don't know what to do. She replies, Maybe a bath with candles, then see if you're hungry, or go and see some friends. Do what your body wants. My body wants a baby and that ain't going to happen yet; not for what seems like far too long a time.

I've managed half a plate of food, an apple and maybe two pints of water all day. It's no wonder I feel sick and exhausted. I've been moody, sad and empty with no idea of what to do with myself. There's a pile of stuff waiting to go into the dishwasher. I can't be bothered with it. The bedroom needs tidying – we're about to run out of clean clothes. It doesn't feel as if any of this stuff matters any more.

I'm not brave enough to pick up the phone. But maybe I don't need to. It didn't take too much out of me to log on to Facebook, and when I did I found heart-warming messages there from friends who're thinking of me. I found a friend request from a complete stranger too. She'd seen our photos, said how devastating they were, but how thankful she then felt that she has all her boys with her. Part of me wants to feel sorry for sharing my photos of Finley. But I don't. If just one person treasures their kids a little more as a result, and gives them a hug for no other reason than that they can, it's been worth it.

Darren phoned while I was in the bath. He's still feeling upset from Monday. He was careful not to mention his daughter Amber, and doesn't want to bring her over to see us, but says we're welcome at their place any time we're ready. According to Darren, Baz and I are both being strong, and were especially brave on Monday. How many more times do I have to tell people: we're not coping; we're barely surviving. There's just no choice.

I am smiling through my tears as I write. It's eleven, and I've only just hung up from a wonderful surprise call with Carolyn and Tania. They asked me what I wanted to talk about, and when I said I didn't know since everything's making me cry or get angry, they went ahead and talked as normal anyway. It's a relief when people behave the same way they always do. I think I might even have laughed. Tania asked the very practical question what are you doing tomorrow? I have agreed to collect the parcel that's been sitting waiting for me at the post office for days. It contains a couple of books by Jason Vale, the Juice Master, since I want to follow a juicing plan. So I'll walk to the post office. It'll give me something to do.

Tania told me about eating for your blood group, so I'll amend my plan to include this. Yes, my plan. It's funny, I'm not interested in losing weight for once; I don't care about that any more. I just want to get a routine going for the coming months. I can't even consider returning to work and am anxious about what will become of my days. Especially when Baz starts work again. The thought of a clear structure brings me some hope. Like putting order into chaos, reason into the irrational. At least it might make some sense of my time.

After the phone call, I checked my emails (if I wasn't addicted to the internet before, I certainly am now). I'd received a couple of quite wonderful messages. The first was from my friend Emma:

```
Hi Mel,

I looked at your photos; the flowers were
beautiful for the funeral and Finley looks very
peaceful. I am glad you had that time with him in
hospital so you have some memories of him to look
back on, even though it must have been unbearably
sad.

I was thinking of you on Monday; on Sunday we all
sat round a candle, and Glyn read Raph's poem which
was beautiful and very moving. I am thinking of you
and Baz a lot and sending light and healing
thoughts. I hope you are managing to get through
the days which must seem very empty. Do let me know
if you ever want a visit or chat.

Lots of love to you both,

Emma xx
```

The second from Alex:

```
You are loved, and you must rest your weary head
and heart on days that feel hard.

Darling Mel, even Superwoman has days when she
takes off her underpants, hides under the duvet and
declares it a day she's incapable of performing
miraculous tasks such as inspiring others. Your
```

leadership, frankness, honesty, compassion, love, humour, is an inspiration to so many.

Rest your head, rest your mind, rest your body; be home, be safe, stay with the love, and leave today and tomorrow to Superman Baz who walks closely by your side.

Reading these, I shed a tear and smiled at the same time. I've often been this way, getting my emotions muddled up. Weeping from laughter or laughing when I'm nervous. Now I'm unhappier than I've ever been and here I am smiling and laughing. And you know what? It's okay. It's actually okay.

It turns out that people want to know how I am but mostly just don't want to intrude. Emma's email has reminded me of this. And Carolyn says people are just waiting for me to give them the word. It's a hard lesson to learn, even now. Just to pick up the phone and ask. But it's coming through loud and clear, especially today. Even if I fear that life goes on for everyone else, I see now that they haven't forgotten us. They haven't forgotten Finley.

To Finley,

Everyone keeps saying your mummy is brave. I don't feel brave. Today I couldn't find the heart or the strength to come and see you, or light your candle. It hurts too much to think of you. I keep trying not to think of you, because every time I do, I get tears in my eyes. I can't cry, because it hurts in my throat and my throat is blocked.

I'm trying not to think of you but I can't help it. You are everywhere. When my mobile has been on a while, a photo of you comes on. You're all wrapped up in your fluffy blanket – the midwife wrapped you all nice and tight with that blanket. Right up to your chin. You have your spotty hat on, so all I can see are your chubby cheeks, and your chin so much like my dad's (so I know it's like mine too). It breaks my heart. You look for all the world as if you will wake up and cry any second. I long to hear you cry.

Day 19

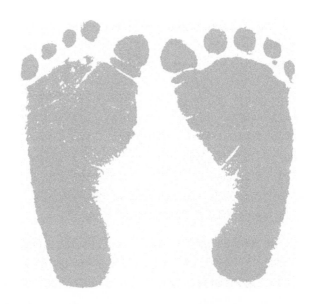

As I walked to the sorting office, the sun was shining. It could almost have been a normal day in a normal life. Except that – all of a sudden – it hit me. The last time I collected anything from the sorting office, I was pregnant with Finley. I was so big I could barely get out of the car. I'd gone to collect a parcel containing a little yellow baby blanket. Recommendations were to buy cellular, not fleece blankets. But I'm so glad now we ignored the advice and got that soft, fluffy yellow one instead. It was perfect for Finley to snuggle up in, smooth to the touch, and soothing to hug him in it and to stroke it. I've always loved that about baby clothes too, shopping for them and feeling how soft they were.

I walked to the town centre post office to collect an application form for Child Benefit. I've discovered we can claim this and that we'll get Child Trust Fund money too. Nobody mentioned it at the hospital. It's a pretty big deal because it means we can put the money towards Finley's gravestone. All of this is proving ever so expensive, and we haven't even seen the bill from the funeral directors yet. We have to pay for the coffin and service sheets, but I don't think there's a fee for the funeral directors' time, or for the vicar or use of the church itself. Mum and Dad paid out for the food, drink and flowers, so that's one to tick off the list. Poor Baz is still distressed about not being able to afford the gravestone. He says it's his responsibility as Finley's dad and he won't give it up. It destroys me to see him in such a state. At least these benefits will be on the way soon. Turns out I've got to phone up to ask for the claim form.

I was supposed to see Barb today, and she'd called while I was out, so I arranged a time and got a lift to the hospital from Baz. He didn't come in with me. It felt important for me to go alone since this was the same hospital we'd been to for most of our antenatal appointments. Also, seeing her without Baz meant I could talk more freely. I didn't have to worry about upsetting him. Look at that, there's me moaning about people pussyfooting around me, when here I am treating Baz with kid gloves.

Barb spent her lunch break with me – an hour and a half at the very least. I really enjoyed it: laughter and tears all the way. I showed her Finley's order of service, and she cried reading Raph's poem. Do we get comfort from the words? Barb asked. I don't know if either of us do. Not right now. It's all still far too raw. Even so, the poem does conjure up a magical image of Finley gliding among the stars. Baz and I love looking up at the stars. When we were in Egypt, we went stargazing in the desert and got some photos of Saturn. We'd taken the trip just after the miscarriage. One of those holidays we always seem to go on – a getaway just after something terrible has happened.

When Barb read the letter I'd written to Finley, she suggested I write a book about our experiences that could help other people in similar circumstances. She was sure other parents of angel babies would benefit from reading about all the choices we'd made, all the ways we'd decided to mark Finley's passing. All those details of how and why we'd created the memories we had in the ways we had.

I don't feel I need to see Barb for my physical well-being any more. My scar has healed and I haven't taken painkillers since Saturday. I'm still bleeding and it's been heavier since Monday. But Barb says that so long as the blood is dark in colour and not offensive, there's nothing to worry about. Blood loss after a caesarean section is much the same as it would be after a natural birth. The womb lining is still being shed and blood loss can continue for up to six weeks in either case. It hardly seems fair to have to put up with such a thing for as long as that. Still, I've been feeling pretty rotten overall, so asked Barb to take a blood test. Of course, I'm hardly eating properly, and my iron levels were very low even before I left the hospital. I need to get checked out.

When Barb asked, I felt clear that I'd like to stay in touch with her. She's been hugely supportive and I like her very much. She has a little boy called Finlay. He's disabled, and I'd love to meet him. On top of that, I want her to be my midwife when I get pregnant again. I told her as much. She was delighted, saying she'd not feel right if someone other than her was to look after me. I'm already talking about getting pregnant again. I can't believe it. But I have a completely overwhelming need to be a mum. I heard someone say it's because all these hormones are still floating around my body, expecting there to be a baby here for me to care for. Barb added that it's not about wanting to replace Finley, just that the need to be a mum is so strong in me.

She promises I'll have a great deal more support next time round. I'll get regular scans and be able to see her as often as I need. Every day if need be. I can pop in for a check-up whenever I want. That's great, although I can't help but think it wouldn't have made an iota of difference in Finley's case. Everything had seemed fine. He'd had a strong heartbeat right up until the final moments. Regular scans wouldn't have changed a thing. Perhaps if I'd had a caesarean earlier, he could have been resuscitated. But I know I'd never have agreed to that without a medical reason for it. And there was none. Oh, how I'd wanted that water birth! I remember sobbing when they told me I needed to be monitored, knowing straight away it meant there'd be no water birth. I mean, I was literally on the verge of going home.

Barb and I also spoke about contraception. Baz and I have discussed it already. I can't even contemplate birth control. I can't bear to think that we might prevent a pregnancy. Another baby's life. It's outrageous in a way I know, but it's a powerful feeling and I won't apologise for it. Medical advice (just like after a miscarriage) is to wait two to three cycles for things to recover and settle. Barb says there's probably little risk. Women can get pregnant by surprise suddenly after a birth and all is well.

The hospital doctor had told me that I wouldn't be allowed to carry another baby to full term, and I questioned Barb about it. I already knew I wouldn't be able to go to the Mackay Birth Centre. Any subsequent labour would be classified as high risk and monitored. Perhaps labour could be induced early? I knew there'd be no water birth this time. And yet, as we talked about it all, I realised that I don't much care how my baby arrives. Nothing I thought was important really counts any more. A caesarean doesn't seem to be the evil it once did (although I'd like it to be performed by the same surgeon if I do have to have one). Even my fear of going into hospital has diminished. Everyone at the hospital was caring and respectful, and my physical well being was a top priority. I had no infection, suffered little pain, and only had one bad day.

All I care about is that my baby is healthy. I want her to be healthy. I want her to be a girl. I do so hope I have a girl. Another boy too soon would be hard to bear. I just couldn't replace Finley.

When I was pregnant with him, we hadn't wanted to know our baby's sex in advance. But we'll definitely need the time to get used to the idea next time round if he is going to be a boy.

I've been ranting so much I've forgotten to mention Finley's donation. The funeral directors collected a total of two hundred and forty pounds at the church. Apparently a hundred people were there on Monday. Adding the seventy we were given makes a total of three hundred and ten pounds. Amazing. Even though it feels like we're the only ones this has happened to, there are hundreds of people around us, friends and strangers, who are being affected. I have almost too many ideas about what to spend the money on. Ideas about what should be available to all parents in the Conway Suite. I told Barb my ideas and she confided in me that she wouldn't have thought of most of them herself. While she understood how vital it was for us to have our time with Finley, she said that only someone who's been through the experience can have real insight into what's needed. So I've arranged to discuss the whole thing with Jill, the bereavement midwife.

My main concern is that most parents of angel babies don't spend as much time in hospital as we did. We had three whole days. It's pretty unusual. It meant I benefited from all kinds of invaluable support and suggestions. It gave us the time to make those memories that are now everything to us. So, I'd like a book or folder of ideas to be placed in the Conway Suite. I want to buy soft, fluffy blankets and teddy bears. Most people won't have the luxury of time to get hold of that sort of thing. They helped me beyond belief. If we get an electric oil burner, it will mean rose oil can be burnt there (rose oil helps in times of emotional stress). Small, individual bottles of baby toiletries should be available too. We'd been forced to use the toiletries used by other parents. Parents with live babies. It upset me terribly to have to do it. I wish I'd had my own, tiny bottles. I could have kept them in Finley's memory box to hold onto those precious memories of giving him his bath, the only Mummy-like thing I'd been able to do with him. Special newborn baby outfits should be hung in the Conway Suite too. It'll give parents the chance to dress their baby in lots of different clothes if they want to.

The Conway Suite should definitely have its own copy of Pat Schwiebert's book We Were Gonna Have a Baby, But We Had an Angel Instead. Other important things, including the equipment to take casts of feet and hands, could be provided. Longer-term mementos, such as pewter casts and jewellery, would be wonderful too. The Colourful Coffins brochure should be prominent. When we were there, the hospital chaplain told us the hospital could take care of everything free of charge. She said little about our other options. But since Mum didn't want us to use the hospital service, we informed them we'd make arrangements with an outside vicar. In hindsight, I'm relieved Mum took charge. The hospital only offers a cremation service. I wonder if parents get told the time and date and if they actually receive their baby's ashes. It turns out that cremations of babies that take place at peak times of day often leave no remains because the machinery is so hot and the body so small.[ii] I was shocked to read this online, and deeply thankful that Mum chose a private funeral, even if it meant we had to pay. It was bad enough signing the release form to authorise removal of the body to the funeral directors. Had we opted for the hospital service, we would never have had that incredible time with Finley at home. Other parents should be given the same chance we did to have special moments like that.

When I spoke to Mum just now, she told me she wants us both to return to work. I guess she's worried we've got nothing to distract us and are getting depressed. But neither Baz nor I are ready to go back. It could be dangerous in Baz's case since he drives a forklift and isn't exactly 'with it' much at the moment. Hell, sometimes it's a trial to get to the shops, let alone even think about spending eight whole hours with other people. I've made the decision to stay away at least until Stephen and Ed have had their babies. We'll be an aunty and uncle twice over in October and I don't know how it's going to affect either of us. No doubt we'll spoil the babies completely. I might be in a state of total grief, but I'll still celebrate other people's happiness. Just like I did when Jade gave birth to Harvey. I was crying as I held him, even though I was over the moon for Jade. Still, I don't think it's a good idea to return to work and then find myself falling apart again come October.

To Finley,

I'm getting used to using your name now. It's so important. You were here, inside me for forty-one weeks and five days. I couldn't give you your name then: we didn't know what type you were! Now this is your name, you should have it and we should use it.

I'm writing with your candle next to me. It is lit and the wax is melting. As the wax goes down, the light of the flame is starting to light up your name. It will be so beautiful when it reaches your picture and you glow with the dancing light of the flame. The candle flame has flickered a lot tonight, even though there's no breeze. It is still now. Maybe you were with me earlier? I hope so. I'll try to walk over to see your grave tomorrow.

Day 20

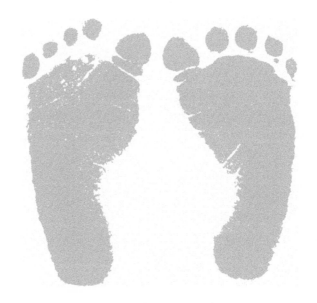

A long, arduous day began when Baz's old workmate Danny told Baz that he and Laura are moving to Liverpool. Laura and the kids are leaving today. We felt miserable saying goodbye, especially after the week we've had. Baz feels he's lost his best friend – Danny is the person Baz sees most in this town. I'll miss Laura too. With three boys, she's a real Supermum. I'll never forget the Christmas we went to their place for dinner. Laura must have presented us with at least seven courses. How she looked after us all so well with a four-year-old running around at her feet and a baby in her arms, I'll never know.

Baz has been really distraught. It upsets me to see him in tears like this. We spent a good deal of the day talking about Finley and what's happened. It's difficult to know whether to feel relieved or overwhelmed that Baz is crying so much. I know there's not much I can do to help. I hadn't realised how much it means to Baz to have a boy. He said he can't help but feel that Finley was his last chance. He wants his son to be a kick-boxer or a footballer. He's been blaming himself too, sensing that he must have done something wrong. So I shared my own anxiety that I hadn't paid enough attention to Finley's movements when he was in my womb. I hadn't known what was supposed to be normal. When I did mention that Finley's movements had changed, the midwife told me they were bound to get less strong as the foetus gets bigger and there's less room for him to move around. Still, it looks like Baz and I are coming to the same conclusion. There was nothing more the hospital could have done. Finley had a heartbeat until the end. We did nothing wrong. I guess we just need to know this for sure.

We went out to Roger and Katy's tonight, for lasagne and a game of cards. They live close by and have been really supportive. Neither of us wanted to go but I'm glad now that we did. We talked about Finley and the funeral of course. Then Katy told us her memories of that first day she'd visited us in hospital. I barely remember a thing. Apparently, I'd called her and she and her girls had been excited to hear my voice. At first. Then they were devastated to get the news that I'd lost Finley. Katy came to the hospital. She was anxious, never having seen a dead body before. But Finley looked as though he was asleep, she said. And he was beautiful. She'd put him into his cot at my request. Neither Baz nor I really remember Katy's visit. But I do recall reading her Facebook status saying 'today I held an angel in my arms'. She'd tended to him just as if he'd been alive. It's exactly what I did. A normal reaction. Natural instinct. It may not have made a difference if Finley had got cold or if his head had been allowed to flop back. But it was impossible not to keep him warm and support his head properly. You just find yourself doing it.

Katy reminded me that the midwife had told us to speak about the baby as if he was alive. This was really important. And while it seemed strange at first, looking back now it's clear – Finley was absolutely alive to us at that point. He was right there, we were still connected, and he felt so close. Had we not stayed in hospital as long as we did, we would have left with barely a single memory of our baby boy. Staying those three days meant we had time to spend with him once the initial shock had worn off. Time we would remember for the rest of our lives.

It pleases me that Katy has asked to see a photo of Finley's coffin, and wants to show it to her girls. They've all seen the photos of Finley on Facebook. I've been getting a bit anxious again about having put photos of a dead baby on Facebook, worrying that people will think it wrong, or weird. But I stop myself. To me, this is a very natural thing to do. I want to show everyone my beautiful baby boy. I want to share him. And I want people to see that there is nothing here to fear. Nothing at all.

I cried again when I talked about Finley to my friend Marie too. Marie believes that all things happen for a reason, and that Baz and I will be parents again in the future. That's comforting, I guess. Already, I can see the positive things that have taken place as a result of Finley's death. But I still wish he hadn't died. We didn't deserve this, Marie said. I can't believe anyone could deserve it.

To Finley,

So many people know you and think of you. You truly are a blessing to me and your daddy. I wish you were here to see all these people who love you.

Day 21

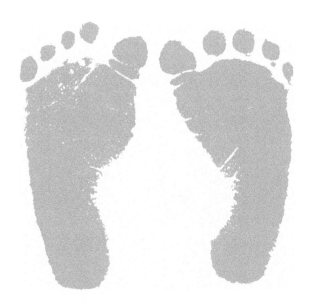

It's been three weeks since Finley was born. That's three weeks I've been wishing I could wake up from this nightmare. Three weeks ago that I was still pregnant and so very excited. Everything's been moving extra slowly today. I didn't get to bed until it was starting to get light. I don't want to go to bed. Night time is the worst. I feel utterly lonely and want to hug Finley and never stop. I have to hug a pillow, or hold Baz really tightly because my arms are gaping and empty. Thoughts upon thoughts race through my mind.

When I'm in bed and Baz is asleep, I think back to the time I was pregnant. I pretend I'm back there. Pregnant again. I'd give anything for it to be true. Even though those last couple of weeks were so uncomfortable. I was in my element when I was pregnant.

Baz and I made love this morning. It was beautiful; it felt so right. But now my mind is off on its travels again. I'm working out when, if I get pregnant, the baby would be due. When we'd be getting the scans done. This is soul-destroying. I simply need to be a mum, that's all.

I've been sleeping on the sofa. Most of the day in fact. All I've managed is to have a shower and drive to see Finley. His grave is only a mile away. I'll easily be able to walk there and back, which will give me something to fill my time. The flowers on his grave are starting to die now, like the flowers at home. That's the trouble with flowers; they die. Everything dies. Then they leave a blank, empty space where they once were. At first it's easy to remember why everything looks so bare. But then, gradually, you start to forget what was there and all of a sudden that cavernous space seems more real than the thing that once filled it. You don't think of it again until you put more flowers in place of the dead ones.

At the cemetery, I found Finley's blue windmill broken, so I fixed it. I've taken away the blue ribbon with Finley's name on it from Tony's flowers, and the badge from the Plymouth Argyle teddy. I've also taken a thistle and a feather that blew across in front of me. I'll put them into Finley's memory box. I've left the teddy that Tony and Liz put on his flowers, it will mark the grave. I don't know what to put on it once the flowers die. It'll just be a patch of empty ground then. Maybe bluebells and snowdrops to mark the end of winter, time moving on. Us moving on.

There's a little girl's grave near Finley's with her photo on it. I'd like that for Finley. No one would be able to forget how beautiful he was. This little girl should have been a year old on Friday. Her family had laid pink helium balloons and birthday cards on the grave. It's devastating to think of reaching such a milestone. Finley's seems far away. What will our lives be like then? I just hope I'm not in so much pain.

Yesterday was the first time Baz and I both had a bad day. We talked and Baz cried when we spoke about Finley. Asked to change the subject. He said he'd told Danny about wanting another baby. When Danny asked him if he'd redo Finley's room for a new baby, Baz said no, Finley's room will stay as it is. It will become the new baby's room as soon as we are blessed to be parents to a baby who stays with us. The baby will play with Finley's teddies, and we will talk about his or her special big brother Finley who left us to look after his big sister or brother. Baz and I agree on all of it.

I must find another way to refer to the days we find the most challenging. Those harder days. I don't want to call them 'bad' days any more. They're not 'bad'. They are what they are, neither good nor bad. They're just days like all the rest. If I say a day is 'bad', then that's how I'll experience it. There are some days when I miss my baby boy so much I am in physical pain. There are days that, when I start to cry, I can't stop. Days I feel so sick I can't eat. They're just days like all the rest.

To Finley,

I wonder if you can hear me when I speak to you at your grave; I don't feel you close to me any more. I went into your bedroom today, but didn't feel you there either. I'm sorry that your grave doesn't have your name on it yet; maybe I can find a door sign to mark it for you?

I'm going to put some wind chimes in your tree. Look after your big brother or sister, and look in on us soon.

I love you my baby boy. You are three weeks old today.

Day 22

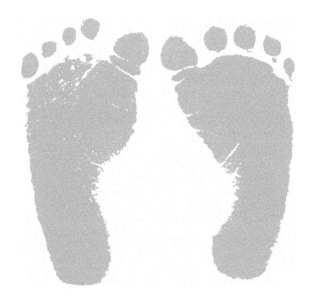

I have nothing to write about. I'm down and I'm grumpy and I simply can't be bothered. Baz is miserable, has a sore stomach and can't be bothered. We've done the shopping and we've eaten. That's pretty much it. Oh, and Baz cooked a stir fry. I've been asleep most of the day. I wasn't tired. I just couldn't be bothered.

Friends have invited us to visit. Mick's asked us to a barbecue in Plymouth this weekend. Matt wants us to go out on Sunday. I don't know how to respond. I'm finding it an effort to think about going anywhere. As though life is threatening to go back to normal and I'm resisting. I'm not ready to let it happen. While I'm sure people aren't expecting us to snap back to how we were before, I really am tired of having to find an answer when people ask, "How are you Mel?" I don't know what to say. How many times can I get away with replying Shit, I'm shit, and it's all just shit? How many times before people get fed up, and tell me to get over it?

Speaking to Nina and Tania has helped me feel better. I told Tania about Finley's flowers dying and leaving an empty patch of earth at his grave. She said that Jewish people don't put flowers on graves but instead mark them with stones. I've taken to the idea. Tania's going to talk to Carolyn and they'll come and lay stones and plant snowbells (snowdrops and bluebells) with me. On Facebook, I confided in Chloë that I struggled yesterday when I couldn't feel Finley at his grave. I couldn't understand it because when we were in hospital and then when we brought him home, he'd felt so close. "He'll be with his sister then", Chloë remarked. I hadn't thought of that. "He'll know you need time and space to heal, and he'll visit you again."

To Finley,

One hundred and four people all around the world confirmed that they had lit a candle for you. Nina told me tonight that her man Greg and his soldier mates who were away at the time lit a candle in the nearest church for you.

You have touched the lives of so many people. You have made big changes for such a little guy.

Love you baby boy. Night night xx

Day 23

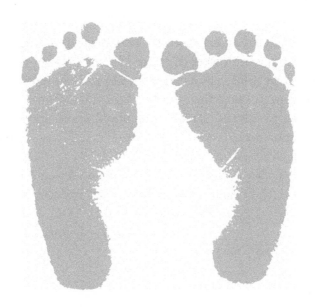

Baz woke me at noon and I got up. An improvement for me but Baz hadn't slept. I'll bet I was snoring! I've started following Jason Vale's Juice Master plan and hope it'll get me eating properly. I've really struggled to put food in my mouth three times in a single day. Even today, all I could manage was half a salad.

Baz helped Danny pack, then we went together to see Finley. Baz does so well – he speaks to Finley out loud. I listened as he reported the football scores. He reckons Finley is cross because Liverpool lost to Aston Villa. Baz wants to get new flowers too now that they're all dying. So we talked about the other things we might do to make Finley's grave look good until we can get him a headstone.

There was a new grave in the cemetery. A little girl. She must be the baby the midwives told Katy about. She died a couple of days after Finley. It's a strange kind of feeling when you think of all the other kids buried there. I hadn't considered how saddened I'd be. Or how distraught it'd make me to know that another baby had died. Two gorgeous flower arrangements were spread over the new grave. One spelled out the little girl's name and the other was a butterfly in pink and purple flowers. There was also a stone angel wearing a necklace. The cards said much the same as ours. No surprises there. I mean, really, what can people say? Baz said he wants to put flowers on all the other kids' graves when it's their birthday because he thinks of them as Finley's friends.

I told Baz I can't feel Finley any more and am devastated about it. Baz confided in me that he doesn't feel Finley with him now either. But it doesn't stop him imagining Finley's replies when he talks to him.

To Finley,

Your daddy and I came to see you today. It was a lovely sunny day. You have a new friend near you. I hope you meet her and look after her. I miss you and love you lots.

Day 24

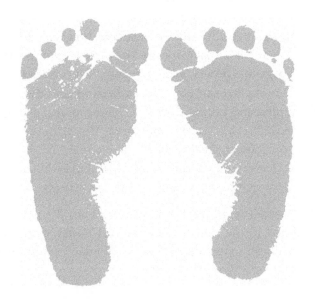

Finley's windmill has broken again but we couldn't fix it. We'll have to get him a new one. I also need to call the cemetery. I'm going to re-sculpt the teddy bear and heart arrangement in silk flowers and need to collect the oasis foam on Friday. So we don't want the gardeners to take away the dead flowers yet. We'll lay some fresh flowers on the grave in the meantime. The snowdrops and bluebells we'll plant next week. And Baz is going to put a flower from us on the little girl's grave.

We were with Finley only briefly since we had to head off to Redditch, Baz driving. We had people to see. Tony and Liz first, then his aunty Renée, for tea. We really wanted to see Baz's cousin Nina and little Zoë before they go back to Germany. Zoë's absolutely gorgeous. Two in January, she's running around and chattering away like crazy.

We watched the videos of Finley on their TV. Zoë whispered night night baby, when she saw him on the screen. The cutest thing. Yet at the same time almost unbearable. So it's mixed emotions for me as ever. I feel joyful being able to show people the videos, to share with them how beautiful Finley is. But it also fills me with sorrow to watch myself in that moment and to know how soon after the filming we'd had to leave Finley in the hospital alone.

To Finley,

We're going to have to get you some indestructible toys – the windmills need to be strong to withstand the wind on that hill. I'm going to put some wind chimes in your tree even if your daddy says they'll annoy you.

I love you so much, you are beautiful. You definitely take after me!

Day 25

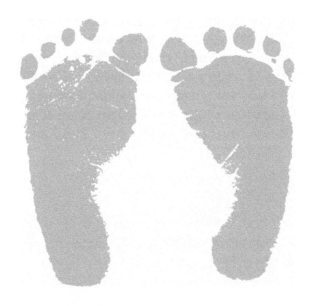

I'm sitting at the computer crying. I've been reading websites about stillbirth and neonatal loss and can't help it. I felt fine earlier and now I'm in a state. I'm still wondering whether or not this is really a very healthy thing for me to be doing right now. Is it possible that I can be crying and still be okay? I mean, I lost my baby less than a month ago. Surely it's normal to be bawling all the time. Yes, crying is a normal part of grief. It says so right here on this site. But it also tells me that the average person grieves for a period of eighteen months to two years. Two years! Surely not! I can't imagine feeling this way for two whole years.

We went to the garden centre and bought a whole bunch of stuff to put on Finley's grave. Now we've got a Winnie-the-Pooh garden ornament and a stone box with In Loving Memory on it. The box will go at the head of the grave and we'll put flowers in it. We've got bulbs, wind chimes and some fresh flowers too. I chose sunflowers as I find them really cheering. At the pub for lunch, I couldn't finish my chicken and salad.

After lunch, we started clearing the dead flowers from Finley's grave. I felt uncomfortable doing it, but you can't keep dead flowers. All that was left was a square of muddy earth with slugs on it. Worse than the empty space left behind when we threw away the dead flowers at home. It reminds me of what happens to everything when it returns to the earth. Not something that's bothered me before. Why would it? I spent a good deal of time on a farm when I was young and thought I had a fair appreciation of life, death and fertiliser. But now it's my baby under there and I can't do a damn thing about it. I can't stop thinking that's my baby there, in the ground. But I've got to try. It's just that it raises so many tough questions. Questions that have a different answer depending on who you ask, or what you believe.

I've collected the oasis foam as planned. Now, there's a stone pot at the head of the grave filled with fresh purple and white chrysanthemums and two sunflowers. A white teddy-bear (from Tony) sits to one side, and Winnie-the-Pooh to the other. In the grass behind that, two windmills. There's snowdrop and bluebell bulbs all dug in at the foot of the grave, with two more sunflowers laid on top of the soil. We didn't lay the flowers and card at the new grave because there were people sitting there. But we did put some pink flowers and a card on a little girl called Mia's grave. It would have been her birthday.

Baz has hung wind chimes in the hawthorn. They're on a fairly low branch, since he didn't want to climb the tree. That concerns me. I mean, anyone could take them. While I was online looking for headstones, I came across quite a few articles reporting that babies' graves are being targeted by vandals. I really am worried that Finley's grave could be vandalised.

Carolyn and Tania have invited me to a retreat. When Carolyn asked me, I completely panicked. I don't know why. I used Baz as an excuse. He wasn't happy and told me as much. On reflection, coming as it had at the end of a day that had seemed so much about moving on, this felt far too strong a reminder that we, too, are moving on. Clearing the flowers because they've died. Going shopping; buying a dress for a wedding that I'd planned to take Finley to. Planting snowdrops that will come up in spring. Knowing that spring will indeed come. That just as the seasons change, so life moves on.

We're off to Plymouth soon. But instead of taking our baby to show off, we'll have to face eyes full of tears, well-meaning hugs, then more and more tears as more and more alcohol is drunk. We'll be out both nights this weekend too. It feels like we're betraying Finley. The simple things are proving the hardest. I know it'll do me the world of good to go to Tania's, but right now I can't even work out how to get there. The arrangements seem beyond me. It'll take four whole hours whatever mode of transport I take. And it's actually proving too much of struggle to concentrate long enough to decide. Being around people, that takes immense concentration too. It's surprising what hard work it is focusing on being okay socially even if it's just for a short space of time. It was a relief to hear from my friend Warren earlier – at least he tells it how it is. So refreshingly untactful.

To Finley,

I dreamt of you last night. I could feel you in my arms. I could feel the way your head fits the shape of my arm perfectly and I could hear your snuffly breathing because you have the same low bridge on your nose as I do. Was I imagining you there, remembering you, or dreaming you could be there? It doesn't matter – you were there.

For three blessed days you barely left my arms. I will treasure the memory of those days and dream of them often.

Day 26

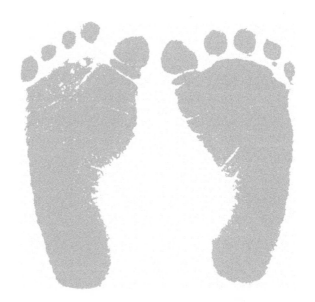

It felt good to be up earlier this morning and go straight out. Mum took me shopping in Weston-super-Mare and totally spoiled me. Truly wonderful. There was a time when I thought I'd never want to go shopping again, so perhaps things are on the up. I came home with brown trousers in a size sixteen, and a cream top with butterflies on it in a fourteen. Add to that a fitted denim jacket in beige, a grey top, black trousers and three pairs of new shoes. I am not kidding! There's a turquoise pair that'll match the top I wore to Finley's funeral. It means I'll get to wear it again. Baz is going to go mad what with all these shoes. Reckon I may have to throw some of my old ones away.

Not only do my new threads look good on me, but I'm fitting into a size smaller than I wore even before I got pregnant. Of course I'm still struggling to eat. So I've not exactly lost the weight in a healthy way. At least juicing has been useful; the juices don't make me feel full and sick like solid food can.

I bought a few bits for Finley. A pot for My First Curl. I have a very fine lock of Finley's hair and have already placed it inside. I'll put the pot in the memory box. I bought a cardholder for Finley's grave, and a book-shaped stone ornament with To My Dear Son and short poem on it. I must remember to write down the verse tomorrow so I can keep it. Mum and I took the lot to Finley's grave, placing the stone book into the ground next to the teddy and Joyce's card into the cardholder. The new little girl's parents were already at the cemetery when we arrived. I was uncertain about whether to say hello. Do we have to be friends just because we're going through a similar experience?

A strange thing happened. I was in the house, bending over to take some chicken out of the freezer. I thought Baz had walked past me and I turned round to check. He wasn't there. He hadn't been anywhere near me, let alone brushing past behind me. Then, Baz thought I was standing by him stroking his head. Again, I was nowhere nearby. It's like we're both being super sensitive right now. I guess grief must open you up to all kinds of new experiences.

Duncan came over this evening. He didn't want to see photos of Finley, didn't feel he was emotionally capable of dealing with it. But he did say he'd like to visit the grave – Baz wants to visit

Finley anyway before we leave for Plymouth in the morning. I must take the camera to get a picture of how it looks now.

We've had a letter from the health visitor offering individual or group support and counselling. I'm not sure what to think. Maybe I'll meet up with her to discuss the options. I don't really think I need to see a counsellor. My lows seem pretty natural to me. I've lost my baby and my dreams are on hold, so I'm obviously going to be miserable. I get angry too sometimes. But it's got to be par for the course. It certainly doesn't mean counselling is the answer. Not right now. Counselling can't change what has happened. It can't bring him back. Still, maybe a support group would work for me. It'd be as much about helping others as helping myself. The thing is, I accept my feelings. I accept the feelings of sadness, loss and grief. The anger, frustration and regret. I accept them all.

I've just had an interesting conversation with Adam, Carolyn's partner. Adam has been quite affected by everything that's happened to Baz and me. I took my time explaining all the different 'spiritual' ideas I've been thinking through, and especially the fact that, because Finley existed, all kinds of positive things have happened. All kinds of healing have taken place. Both within me and in the world around me. Adam felt this was all a continuation of the work I've been doing on myself in recent years. I've done a lot of it – in courses and in my own daily practice – and I now have all sorts of techniques that support my personal development in my day to day life. The experiences with Finley have brought this to a whole new level. And right now, I feel very very thankful for Finley and all that he has given us.

To Finley,

I am so grateful you chose us to be your parents. I am blessed to have known you, in the way that only I could. I am so happy to have found the peace I have been searching for, for such a long time.

I am so glad we had nine months when it was just you and me. I know you, and I know all you are. I know all you are and I love all you are.

Day 27

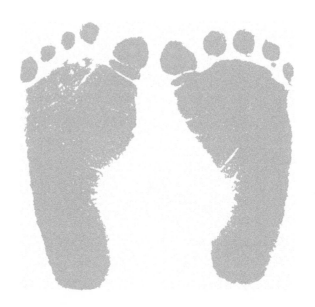

We were late getting up today, but still had time to take Duncan to see Finley. His windmill has broken again! We really do need to get a new one. Someone has put wind chimes on the grave of the twins nearby. They're attached to little wooden stilts like flat bird-boxes. I put the card and flowers down on the little girl's grave.

Once in Plymouth, we went straight to see Matt, Leanne and Jason. Gemma was there too. Matt will be DJ-ing a cheesy music set on Sunday so we trawled through his CDs for fun tracks. We had a real laugh – he's got some hilarious stuff. Baz demonstrated his usual lack of good taste by playing the 'Star Trekking' song and singing along with it. There were some pretty gloomy moments too: I played Cats in the Cradle which has the line 'when you coming home son, I don't know when we'll be together'.

Gemma chose Stand by Me for Baz and me. She was looking at photos of Finley at the time and it reminded me how beautiful I'd thought the black and white photos would look as a slide-show set to music. Gemma ended up seeing all the photos we've got on the camera, even of Finley in his coffin. I hadn't meant for her to see them – no one else has yet. She sobbed out loud.

We didn't stay long at the barbecue Beverley and Mick. Baz was struggling to explain everything to so many people, and to reply to the rounds of 'how are you?' And 'are you okay?' We left early and had a game of poker and lots to drink at home. Beverley and Mick don't have a single photo of Finley yet. So we really need to get them copies. The picture of Finley's scan is under a lamp with a card saying 'Big Hugs'. I don't think Beverley's coping well with this. I think she feels too far away from her son. Mick said he was proud of Baz. I'm proud of him too. He's an incredible husband and will be a superb father too. As soon as he gets the chance.

To Finley,

The impact you've had on our lives extends far beyond our little corner of Bridgwater. Your Nana Taylor and Gramps love you very much. Gramps had to go to a job interview the day after we said hello and goodbye to you. He couldn't concentrate and didn't get the job. I hope you're watching over him and find him the perfect job.

Day 28

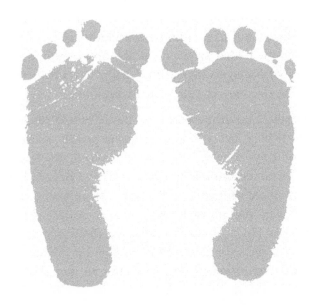

I usually hate Bingo. Last time I went I was pregnant, and so distracted by my raging hormones and squirming tummy that I missed the fact I'd won. Twice. Today, at Beverley and Mick's social club, I won three lines and two houses. Pity there weren't more people there. I only won around twenty quid, but it paid for a few drinks. Baz won the stand-up, adding twelve more.

Leanne and I went out dancing. I got really drunk, but managed to carry on dancing for a good while. I enjoyed myself. It was great to feel like any other normal person. Just for a bit. I kept wanting to talk to people about Finley and everything that's happened. One minute I was yelling I'm making the most of the drink – I haven't had one for nine months. Next thing, all I wanted to say was Stop, people! My baby died! Why are you all having a good time?

Jo and Phil were out on the town too. As operating department practitioners, they were keen to ask questions about Finley. I'd asked the same questions myself, of course. Exactly the stuff I'd been unable to get out of my head. Could anything have been done differently? What if I'd done this or that? Mentioned this or that? Asked for this or that. Could they have been any different? It's easy to drive yourself mad thinking about things like that all the time. None of it's going to change a thing.

Jo and Phil were concerned that the doctors had been too late carrying out the caesarean. I defended the doctors; they couldn't have done otherwise, and they did the operation in just ten minutes. It wasn't so much the operation itself, Phil said, but the timing of their decision which could have made a difference. Phil couldn't let go of the idea that we'd been failed somewhere along the line. Of course you have been failed, he told me. You have a dead baby. He was so blunt it stopped me in my tracks. Our baby is dead and we don't know why. Maybe it'd be better to know, even if we do beat ourselves up about it. Even if we do find out we didn't protect him properly. Mind you, I'm doing that anyway. I have a mother's guilt even though I'm not a mum.

I've been preparing a list of questions for the midwife and doctor, so it's been helpful to have this input. I've probably been getting far too caught up in how thankful I am for the care I received after the birth. And not wanting to upset the wonderful staff who helped us in the Conway Suite.

Day 29

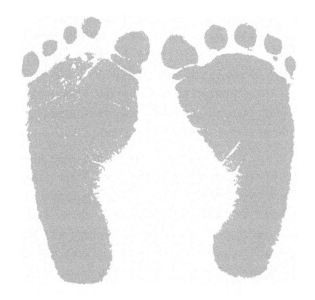

Bank Holiday Monday and I've been sleeping off a hangover for most of the day. Why do we do it to ourselves? Still, the alcohol seems to have stimulated my appetite. I've eaten twice. What an achievement!

There's something wrong with Baz. Maybe a bug. It's definitely not just a hangover. He's not likely to be going back to work quite yet. He'll be here with me for a few more days and I'm glad. I've become quite clingy. Of course, we could do with the money. We've booked a room with a four-poster bed and Jacuzzi bath for the weekend of Joanne and Duncan's wedding. I hope we can still go. I must remember to phone the hotel to tell them we don't need the cot we'd requested. That's going to be tough. The money issue pales in comparison.

Like it or not, the wedding's going to be rough for me. There'll be more sympathetic glances and offers of shoulders to cry on. People making sure we're okay. Only a few months back, I'd been looking forward to all the congratulations, all the minor quarrels over who'd get to cuddle my baby first. I'd imagined taking Finley there dressed in a cute little outfit. Instead we buried him in one. Instead of lounging on the four-poster bed feeding my baby, I'll be drinking enough to get me through the emotions of the day and make sure I'm drunk enough to sleep that night.

Baz and I were already talking about trying for a baby the last time Joanne tied the knot. It was just before we got married ourselves. Now Joanne's divorced and almost married again and still we have no baby.

Day 30

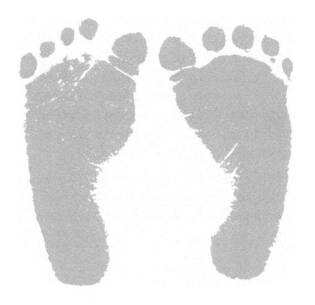

I woke up at two in the afternoon, Baz still tucked up beside me. He must be ill. He never stays in bed and hasn't been sleeping properly during the night. So I let him sleep in some more. When he woke up at last, he phoned the doctor to make an appointment to ask for a sick note. He'd be expected at work tomorrow otherwise. No way he's ready for that yet – he'd be a liability.

The doctor made my blood boil. He didn't even remember Baz, so the poor thing had to explain everything that's happened all over again. He came out with a sick note for two more weeks and a prescription for Temazepam on account of the lack of sleep. Not even an offer of grief counselling. What's a GP doing prescribing an addictive drug to someone with a history of depression and drug misuse? I guess he did only prescribe two weeks' worth, so that must make it alright. Forgive the sarcasm.

I'm putting my better mood and energy levels it down to the juicing, so popped out for more fruit and vegetables. It really is so much easier to juice than eat. We picked up my dress for the wedding from Mum too. It's an Empire line in three vivid shades of blue chiffon. The flattering cut skims over my belly and makes my boobs look great. And the charm necklace Carolyn gave me is the perfect colour to match. It has a silver crescent moon charm with a child sitting on it, a blue glass heart, and a grain of rice with Finley's name on it set in a tiny vial of water.

The dress is a size sixteen and looks really good, but it's clear I could've got away with a fourteen. It's the second time in a week I've noticed this and I'm still shocked by the way the weight's been falling off. Still, I can honestly say that I'm starting to feel comfortable with my body for the first time in a very long time. It's as though all those issues that were tied up with the abuse I suffered at the hands of my ex-boyfriend are starting to dissolve. The fear has gone.

The experience of pregnancy has been part of that process. It's truly amazing to conceive, carry and give birth to a baby. You look at the body in a whole new way. I so hope I get to experience it again. The stretch marks, though – those I could do without. They only appeared in the last two weeks of pregnancy, can you believe it? Nine months and then ... eek!

Jill's coming over tomorrow. I'm going to ask her the questions I've prepared. I know the bereavement midwife visits every couple that loses a baby, so she's bound to be used to all those questions beginning with Why...? We're seriously going to need to tidy up this bomb-site of a house before she gets here as I haven't done a scrap of housework all week.

I'll also talk to Jill about the contribution we want to make to the ward. I've decided to set up a charity in Finley's memory and donate a cold cot to the Conway Suite. A cold cot would give parents the chance to spend more time with their baby, just as we did. It's basically an ordinary hospital cot with a motor underneath so that the base is maintained at a temperature of zero degrees. This way, the baby's body is kept cold and doesn't change as quickly as it otherwise would. I'm not sure whether or not they've got a cold cot at the hospital already. Finley's body did go quite cold. On second thoughts, I'm sure it would have stopped his nose bleeding if they'd used it. I'd have welcomed that.

To Finley,

We are meeting Jill tomorrow, and we will be able to see the notes from the morning you were born. I hope we find out what happened to you.

I like to think that you had chosen not to stay, and that this was not your time. I hope there was nothing we could have done to change the outcome. If there was and I had known at the time, I would have done it. I would have done anything to take you home in my arms.

Day 31

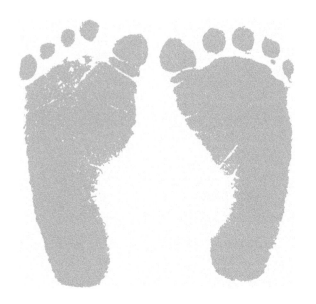

I'm feeling guilty for not going to see Finley. I wanted to stay strong for Jill's visit. The prospect of asking all these questions – questions I need to know the answers to – made me very nervous. At first, we talked about what I intend to do with the money we've collected from the funeral and since. There's now three hundred and fifty pounds to buy things for the Conway Suite.

I've made some adjustments to my original list of items. Fluffy blankets are a dead cert, but we need smaller ones than the one we had for Finley, especially for babies born very early. I'm still keen on getting a range of baby outfits as well as the wonderful We Were Gonna Have a Baby, But We Had an Angel Instead. It's a great book for helping remove the fear and stigma around stillborn babies. It also allows parents to talk to their other children in simple terms about what's happened, encouraging them to spend time as a family with the baby. I want to include a whole bunch of other story books for babies too, so that people have the chance to read to their baby if they so choose. Miniature individual toiletries that people can take away with them are a must, and we'll display a note along with them saying it's okay to bath your baby if you want to. I'm going for the footprint casts too, the electric aromatherapy oil burner (with rose oil to help calm the emotions), some memento cards and pots. I still want the teddy bears as originally planned, but will include one that doubles as a comforter blanket and can be pinned to make a pouch for those tiny little babies who are born too soon.

I explained to Jill why these things are important and how they can help people in situations similar to ours. I want to make sure there are as many options as possible for parents to make their own memories, bond with their baby, and feel reassured in their choices. I want them to know that what they're doing is perfectly normal.

Simple things can prove absolutely vital. Like that extra-fluffy blanket we'd been so lucky to have, helping us feel connected to Finley. Helping us grieve. Blankets provided by the hospital have been used by other parents whose babies are fine. So when you're forced to use a hospital blanket, you can easily start thinking about all the things those other parents are likely to do with their babies that you'll never be able to do with yours. And a soft blanket makes all the difference because it encourages you to hold and stroke your baby. In retrospect this was absolutely essential for me. To be allowed to feel and express that powerful maternal instinct. I took the same blanket home for comfort, and was able to use it to cover Finley's coffin and keep him warm.

So we'll provide things that will help diminish people's fear and give them the freedom to express their natural parental instincts. People still have the same instincts when their baby is stillborn as they do if she or he is living. That's why we'll hang up a small wardrobe of smart baby outfits in the suite. It will encourage parents to take photos with their baby, even keep hold of an outfit their baby has worn as a memento. Dressing the baby in something special is a very different experience to dressing him in clothes bought before he was born. It gives people memories which in some ways are happy ones. Not regrets or more wishes that will never be granted. It also gives parents the chance to actually dress their baby. It might be their only opportunity. Even if they don't feel capable of dressing their baby, they'll have the option of selecting an outfit, which can be just as helpful.

For me, reading Finley a bedtime story really enabled me to bond with him. To do a Mummy thing with him. It meant I'd chosen my last memory of Finley and that it was a happy one. With a small library of storybooks for babies in the Conway Suite, other parents will get that same chance. If they want to read their baby a story, they'll be reassured that it's an acceptable thing to do. There should never be any judgement or stigma involved when parents want to spend precious moments with their baby after he's dead. It makes me weep buckets to think about it. It was everything to me to know that my feelings were normal and that what I wanted to do was considered acceptable. I desperately needed to know that there was nothing wrong with reading a story to my sleeping baby. That there was nothing more natural than wanting to do so. Now, Baz and I have videos of these last moments and, devastating as they are, wouldn't be without them for the world.

I really like the idea that people can take home the miniature baby toiletries to keep as mementos. Perhaps in a memory box. You know, the strangest things can become important memories. The footprint casts, memento cards and pots (like the one I've put

Finley's hair in) will be in the suite for similar reasons. Teddy bears too. When you have a baby, you expect people are going to buy you presents. But you may well find that nobody does. This is one thing that upset me the most when we got home from hospital. No presents. No teddies or toys. Just white sympathy cards. Nothing at all that said Congratulations on your baby boy.

When you lose a baby in the way we did, you're still full of all your expectations, hopes and dreams. You need more than anything for your baby to be acknowledged as a baby and not swept under the carpet out of fear. Our baby was born and he was here. And he should have some presents. Now the Conway Suite will have its own collection of teddy bears for parents to give to their baby as a present. It's comforting to cuddle a soft toy, and to know that your baby once touched it. It certainly helped me feel closer to Finley. Midwives can suggest taking photos of the baby with a teddy too. I wouldn't want to imagine the guilt you might feel if you hadn't had the chance just to give your baby a teddy bear while you could. You really do need to feel you've done everything you can for your baby.

Jill and I also talked about the cold cot. She thought it was a good idea, making it more acceptable for parents to spend that much needed extra time with their baby. Since physical changes occur more slowly if the baby is kept cool, a cold cot can help diminish fear too. Jill was grateful for all my suggestions and adamant she couldn't have thought of half the things I have. Dealing with cases like ours, she told me, is always a rewarding part of the job since people are so grateful. But it's also upsetting for staff, especially when they're not sure if they're saying or doing the right things. So they want as much feedback as they can get.

Far too soon, the time came for me to ask Jill the questions I dreaded. Here they are., and what I remember of the answers.

1. Why wasn't a caesarean section performed when I'd asked about the baby's movements getting less strong?

a) Jill explained that as babies get to full term they have less room to move, so I would inevitably feel less defined movements, and would have noticed even fewer because I was having light contractions. The machine showed movements so there was no need for concern. The three movements I'd marked down coincided with those the machine picked up. It was all normal.

2. Was a student or agency midwife on the antenatal ward?

a) A fully trained midwife was there.

3. Did the heart rate drop with each contraction at 4–6 a.m.? Why wasn't a caesarean section conducted then, and why didn't they use an internal monitor?

a) The heart rate dropped with one contraction. The problem was not clear, and once it did became clear, the caesarean was conducted quickly. An internal examination was carried out prior to ultrasound, but my cervix was not open so an internal monitor couldn't be used.

4. Why did they perform an ultrasound scan?

a) They performed an ultrasound to check Finley's heartbeat.

5. Did cardiology or placenta problems show?

a) He had a heartbeat, but it was 50 – 60 bpm.

6. Did he have a heartbeat on the ultrasound scan?

a) He had a heartbeat; if he had already died, I would not have had a caesarean section.

7. How many staff are on the antenatal ward at night? Was it busy?

a) It was not too busy, and the midwife stayed with me.

8. Was someone else in theatre?

a) No.

9. What time did the doctor see me on the ward?

a) I can't remember Jill's answer.

10. Why wasn't the caesarean section carried out when I told them the meconium had got thicker and darker?

a) This was at the same time there were problems with the monitor, so they started to check and stayed with me then.

11. Will the coroner be involved with the post-mortem?

a) No.

12.What is the risk assessment panel?

a) When any baby dies, an incident form is completed. The incident is considered by a risk assessment panel to see if any lessons can be learnt from it.

13.Can I find out what is said by the panel?

a) This information is not shared with the public, unless requested.

14.If a caesarean section had been performed earlier, would Finley be alive?

a) Jill feels that there may have been no reason to perform a caesarean section earlier, as Finley's heart rate had risen.

15.Was Finley ill?

a) This is not known.

16.Why were his lips dark in early photos and when Baz saw him?

a) The extremities – lips, fingers, toes – change colour very quickly when the heart stops beating. Often this is the only sign in photos of stillborn babies that they are dead, not sleeping.

17.When I am pregnant again, what care will I have? Can I have a natural birth?

a) Jill repeated what Barb had told me: I'll be able to have whatever I need to keep me as calm as possible through the next pregnancy. I'll be carefully monitored after twelve weeks since Finley was over full term. The doctor would prefer to perform a caesarean section. There's a low risk of my scar rupturing. Jill says she wouldn't carry out an induction as the risk to the baby becomes higher with the introduction of some of the chemicals involved; but it may be possible to have a drip. The best compromise would be to set a date for a caesarean section, but wait to see what happens if I do go into labour naturally prior to that date. I don't know what I think. I just want me and my baby to be safe and well. It says in my notes that I had a uterine inversion. I'll have to ask the consultant about that.

18.Did they try to resuscitate Finley?

a) They have a set procedure of steps, and they tried them all.

Day 32

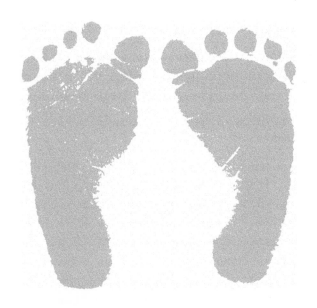

On the whole, I've been feeling alright since Friday, and today's been good too. I went to Katy's for lunch. Her daughter Jacqui is going to colour my hair. I so want that blue colour in my hair! Baz thinks I've gone daft, but the way I see it, I have time to play now. I'm not expected back at work until March, so I don't have to be responsible!

Danni brought her baby Isabelle (Katy's granddaughter) over and I had a cuddle. It felt fine. I reckon other people are more concerned about me seeing babies than I am. I still look forward to the day when I'm a mum to a baby who stays here. I need to be a mum. I need to hold my baby in my arms, see the colour of its eyes and hear its giggles. But that doesn't change who I am – I'm always going to be happy for people blessed enough to have children or get pregnant.

When I got home, Nicola came over. We've known each other since school. She gave me a photo frame. Our house is going to be filled with photographs! We already have three large frames to go on the walls, and two more that'll stand on the shelves. We really are going to have to choose the photos for them pretty soon. I still don't have any photos of Finley on display yet. I can't decide whether or not it'd be best to keep them away in his room, with the door shut, so I can look at them when I want to and not have to see them all the time.

Nicola's been trying for a baby just a little longer than we have and is starting in vitro fertilisation. She didn't want to upset us, talking about it. It really is fine – I'll be happy for her if it works. Hopefully we won't be too far behind with baby number three. And this time our baby will choose to stay with us.

I spoke to Mum about the answers I'd received from Jill. Mum thinks it's helped, because I sound better. She was concerned I was feeling a bit resentful on Tuesday. I wasn't exactly bitter, but I had felt pretty fed up after that conversation with Phil and Jo. It had really got me thinking. I told Mum that I think that the hospital did all they could, as quickly as they could. I may have been a bit economical with the truth there though. I mean, I now know that if they'd performed the caesarean sooner, Finley would be alive. His heart rate was strong. But, because his heart rate was strong, there'd been no reason for them to do the caesarean. In fact, if they'd asked me at that point, I doubt I'd have let them go ahead. A strong heart rate means he wasn't in any distress. So the only point in question is whether another person in another hospital would have performed that caesarean earlier on. I've spoken to my best friend Nadine about this. In her job as an operating department practitioner, she's assisted in lots of emergency caesareans but has never seen one carried out purely because there's meconium in the waters. She also agrees that the presence of meconium does not equal foetal distress. In fact, she's seen many women with meconium in the waters go on to have healthy babies.

I finally spent some time in Finley's room. When I say it out loud, I still say the baby's room. As if it was never his. As if we always knew he wouldn't go into his room. I unpacked the bag of Finley's clothes we'd brought home from hospital, held the clothes he'd worn, and remembered him. One vest has blood on it from his belly-button, as they did not clamp it. I emptied the memory box, very slowly putting back into it all the mementos I'd gathered together. I put the newspaper announcement in the bottom, then on top of that the card from the hospital with Finley's photos, his hand and footprints, and the cards from all the funeral flowers. The presents from Jade are in there too, with the clothes on top. It's jam-packed. I must remember to add the pot with Finley's hair. I sobbed a little as I packed it all up, but I felt good too. It really is good to remember Finley in this way.

I've written a thank you card to the funeral directors:

Thank you for all you did to support us at the most difficult time. The kindness, compassion and flexibility you showed helped us so much. The funeral was beautiful and we did not have any extra stress to deal with thanks to your organisational skills. All the suggestions you made helped us to decide what we wanted.

We are so pleased with the coffin and with the fact that we brought Finley home for the night. The information you gave us and your professional approach helped us do it even though we were anxious. It gave us those precious few hours more with our son. Yours cannot be an easy job but you did it with a comforting smile throughout.

Tomorrow is our friends' Leon and Lorraine's wedding. They're getting married in the same church we did. The same church where we had Finley's funeral not much more than two weeks ago. I hope I'll be okay.

To Finley,

My primary school teacher has died. She was a wonderful teacher — I hope you meet her.

Day 33

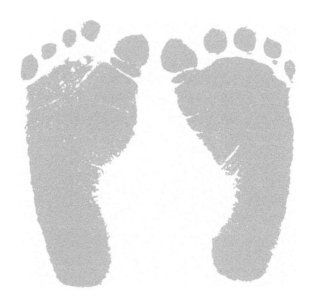

Lorraine made a beautiful bride. She and Leon had a stretch mini as their wedding car and it really made me smile. I'm happy for them – they had a wonderful day. Baz and I managed pretty well all things considered, and I got the chance to hand over our thank you card to Martin, the vicar. The reception was a bit of a trial, though, and we didn't stay too long. I find I really have to be on guard in social situations, and it takes a good deal of concentration to hold it together in front of other people for extended periods of time.

So I met Mum from work and went over to hers. She'd had some of the photos developed from the CD we'd given her. I browsed through them and was fine, but cried when Mum looked at them. It all snowballed a bit then, as Mum got upset because I'd got so upset. I also noticed how angry Dad seems. I suspect he's grieving and feels he can't talk to anyone about it. I think it may have taken him by surprise to discover how much he was looking forward to being a granddad. Dad's family didn't think it important enough to come to Finley's funeral. To add insult to injury, friends of ours had cared enough to travel all the way down from London for the day. Dad's used to being in control, and certainly to being able to help me out. He was in the army for years, so he's no stranger to challenging situations. But this is one situation not even he can change.

I am discovering a strength and clarity that I have started to express to others. I shared this today on Facebook, saying:

At the moment I am being in what perhaps should be the most painful present others can imagine. Yet I am peaceful, at peace, and feeling acceptance and gratitude. I have chosen this route, and choose to be here in this present moment to experience it.

My soul mission may not always be clear; however, I know I am following the path it sets.

I am sure that these experiences will help others in time. I don't know how, nor do I need to. I am here and that is there, and I will find my way there. Of this I am sure.

Day 34

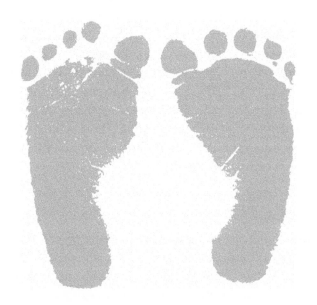

I've felt emotional from the moment I woke up. I'm bleeding fairly heavily and don't know whether to be worried or not – I don't know what's considered normal. Nothing in my body feels normal any more. At the shops, I found myself being unusually short-tempered with Baz, too.

Baz chose some extra-special, extra-large lilies to take to Finley's grave. Next time we'll bring water to see if they last longer. We've also got a pair of scissors stashed in the car now should we need them. All that's left of Finley's windmill is the stem in the ground. Such a shame. We spotted a new potted plant on his grave that neither of us had put there. It had tiny pink flowers on it and a little card too. Inside the card is written:

To Finley,

Please look after Imogen for us until we can be with her again. I'm sure you will be friends and play together. Until then, look after each other. Sweet dreams.

From Imogen's Mummy and Daddy xx

I broke down when I read the card because that's just what I'd want for our babies too. I have a feeling we may end up friends with Imogen's parents after all. They seem to feel exactly the way we feel. They've added some decorative butterflies on stakes to Imogen's grave, and have a solar-powered light shaped like a fairy. A really sweet idea – at least the babies won't be in the dark now.

The autumn leaves have started to fall on Finley's grave, a reminder to me that soon it will be colder and darker. I don't much like the idea of the frosty winter months, the ground being hard and icy and my poor baby being in that frozen earth. The soil on Finley's grave has started to sink. If the caretakers put more soil on it, I'm not too hopeful the snowdrops and bluebells will break through come spring.

Liz gave me a beautiful gift – a ring with a green peridot heart setting. The heart fits perfectly into the gap between the stones of another ring of mine which I bought on Nadine's suggestion last year after my miscarriage. The ring has three aquamarine stones (the birthstone for March). They're set in such a way that – to my eyes – they resemble the silhouette of an angel. When I first bought it, the three stones represented our family; one stone each for me, Baz and our baby. I used to wear it below my wedding band. But now I'm going to put it on the other hand, with the new stone for Finley set snugly in.

Baz is really fuming right now. He just can't believe there's a God because no God would have taken Finley away from us. He's angry that the doctors didn't do the caesarean section earlier. He's hurting too because it's going to be the anniversary of his friend Johnny's death in a few days' time. He says he'll ask Johnny to look after Finley. We talked about it all and had a big hug.

Day 35

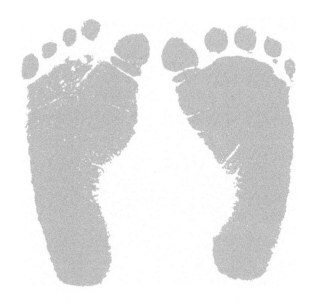

Things have been quiet what with Baz making up for lost sleep most of the evening. I have a lonely feeling inside even though I love getting to spend so much time with him. More time than we've spent together since the three weeks we were on honeymoon in Zante. I definitely don't want him to go back to work yet. We'll manage financially. My hope of an extra income and a safety net stashed away can go on hold for now. Still, my dream for the future is becoming more clear. I want our little family to live in a cosy, old country house with large fireplaces. It will be perfect for me, Baz and our future son and daughter. We'll have land with our own little piece of woodland on it. There, I'll build a special place for people to come and stay, to attend meetings and courses to learn about health and peace. We'll have pigs and lambs so our children can have just the kinds of experiences I had when I was growing up. We'll enjoy flexible work and fewer hours, and generate a good portion of our income passively. That'll give us the time to enjoy our family as well as foster kids who aren't as lucky as our own.

I feel less sad today. As though I'm empty of emotion. I'd thought I was coming down with a heavy cold yesterday, but there's no sign of it. It occurred to me that my physical well-being may well be changing according to my emotional state. This certainly makes sense. I've been receiving some wonderful messages from a woman on Facebook that are definitely related to this train of thought. I'm going to give them more time as soon as I'm feeling less numb. Her messages are odd, a bit mystical and mysterious, fatalistic almost, and it'd be far too easy to adopt a sceptical attitude towards what she says. I can see myself already applying too much logic, rationalising this crazy talk. And I don't think that's helpful. Not here. Not now. You see the thing is, I get this really strong sense somehow that these messages are very significant for me. They're definitely linked to my recent line of thinking about Finley, and to the beliefs I've started constructing around how and why he came to us. But I'm finding it hard to do anything other than just scribble them down here for now. For future reference. I'll have plenty of time to think about all this in the days – and sleepless nights – to come.

My new friend has entitled her first message Lessons in store for you. She writes:

He is still with you, being held and loved by you. He is fine, just as he was before birth. He is enjoying heavenly moments with you by his side. To him this was just a very brief visitation, meant as a wake-up call for you.

Stay together with him in your thoughts; always remain positive. Once you have mastered the level of remaining positive you can guide your thoughts and feelings deeper and deeper, until you come to the essence of truth about the cycles of life.

You are surrounded by angels who take very good care of all of you. Don't be sad. It distracts from the lessons your boy is teaching you. He is a very evolved soul. When you lose your sadness, the divine purpose behind these circumstances will be fully and joyfully revealed to you. Do not cry idle tears. Rewards are greater than what the eye meets now.

Celebrate the gift of your wedding and be very thankful for the love surrounding you. Learn your lessons so you can, in later days, enjoy the new addition coming to your family.

Do not let mind limit you to the earthly world. Nothing, nothing ever happens by accident. A divine purpose will be fully revealed. Know that you are very much loved. You are never alone. Heaven is a safe place, comprised of angels and infinite love.

I tell her I'm not sure I can respond to her message yet but would like to talk about it another time, if that's alright. I am meeting lots of fantastic people on the internet who have different beliefs to the ones I thought I held and that have been changing so much over the past couple of years. Beliefs that appeal to me more and more. I am learning a great deal, and attracting to myself the things I need to learn. I tell this woman I am certain she is a part of this. But that I'm not yet ready to give her ideas the attention they deserve. That I'm too quick to apply logic right now and feel so numb after the emotional intensity of yesterday. I tell her how distressed Baz was, then my mum the day before that. I've had to protect myself today and regroup.

She soon sent me a second message, quite brief. It read: Coincidences will guide you to the right path. Attached was a link to the music video for Bob Marley and Gilbert Gil's Three Little Birds. It's a funny little animation. I must show Baz. I tell her she's making me smile with her intriguing messages and the uplifting video. I say that although I've never been interested in coincidences, at the moment there are so many of them and they are so blatant that I can't ignore them any more. I have time now to open myself wide, immerse myself in freedom. See what comes.

My new friend's reply has touched me deeply and moved me to tears. She's attached a link to the video of Bobby Mcferrin's Don't Worry Be Happy:

You are very loved. God never leaves any of his children down. You are a treasured child of God. Trust in what the heavens are bringing about for you. Follow the coincidences and strange events in your life. This will reconnect you.

Enjoy your marriage. Before long you will have learned the most joyful lessons. Be open to new experiences, the heavens are with you.

There is a very very very happy baby wiggling about here; he needs you to know he is with you and very happy. You are very very very very very loved (very appears forty-two times in the original email). Sorry, that last sentence was written by your son. I kindly had to ask him if this was enough verys for you to get the message: he wanted to put a zillion verys there. The chap is happy and is sending you happiness. Namaste.

So I replied, finally:

Collect the diamonds that are falling from my eyes and landing on my smile and pass them on to Finley for me.

PS. I will not question this message at all – I used to tell him I loved him a zillion times bigger than the sky during my Reiki sessions in pregnancy.

Oh, and the words child of God are not words I would use naturally at all, but they are in a song I treasure from a personal development course I went on. I sang it to Finley often; I sang it to him when he was sleeping in his coffin in his cot; and when his daddy carried him into the church at his funeral.

Blatant coincidences – just need reassurance I am not bonkers. I have worked in mental health for ten years and if my patients told their docs the things that have happened to me recently, they'd be sectioned for being delusional.

To Finley,

Thank you for the message you sent. I love you a zillion times too. I am glad you heard the song I used to sing you. The words are meaningful to me, and now they will be even more so as it will feel like you sing it to me.

I am glad you are happy, and I am smiling as I imagine you wiggling about. You used to wiggle around so much inside of me – Mitsicat was very confused. You once booted your daddy in the side of his head when he lay down on you. We laugh about that.

Mitsi and Gizmo want to go in your room and sit outside it often. When we let them in Gizmo lies at the top of your cot and won't let us pick him up to get him out. I'm sorry we have not been to see you today, I'm sure you want to know the football results.

Day 36

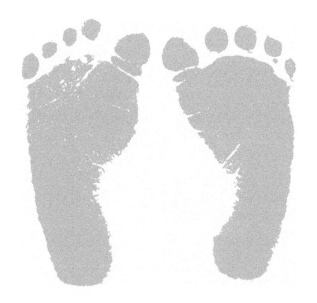

I have no idea what day it is. I've missed my doctor's appointment. Right day, wrong time. I've re-booked for tomorrow. I'll be taking a list of questions because I know I'll forget what I need to say otherwise. My own doctor won't be there as he's recuperating after an operation. He won't know what's happened until he gets back. We used to work together and I know he'll be saddened by my news.

I had a call from my old friend the family therapist. It's helped no end. Put my mind at rest. He says there's an average time to pass through all the stages in the grief cycle, but that some people pass through the cycle more quickly than others. He suspects this time difference could be related to the period for which people are bonded to the person they've lost. Interestingly, the stages don't necessarily come in the same order for everyone, and it's quite normal to pass backwards and forwards between them. He confirmed too that all the things we'd done in the hospital and with the funeral would have helped us move through the grief cycle. I knew we'd been doing the right things – we'd taken our one and only chance to experience what we wanted with Finley and to honour our feelings. It was all part of the process of accepting that he was dead. I knew it then, trusting that what I needed to do was absolutely normal and natural. And I know it now.

Finley had a job to do and he has done it, I explained, feeling more and more clear as I said it out loud over the phone. Just look at what has changed as a result of Finley's being here. Just see what things are 'better' – is that the right word, I wonder? I'm no longer scared of my ex-boyfriend. I'm closer to my parents, more connected with them. I sense a deep peace within me and am no longer full of sorrow. I don't have a problem with my body any more – there's no psychological anguish at all. I am grateful that being pregnant with Finley has allowed all this and more to come to pass.

Everything is perfect, my friend replied, though he doubted perfect could be the right word in the circumstances. But you know what, I really do know what he means. I think that this is the way it was meant to be. I remember having similar thoughts after the miscarriage. I remember thinking that perhaps I had lost that baby so that I could fully accept my need to be a mum. To know how was important it was to nurture myself and my next baby. Perhaps that was part one of this healing process. Perhaps what has happened now is the second stage. When I was pregnant with Finley, I didn't have a single doubt about wanting to be a mum. I know now without a doubt that I would have been a fantastic mum. This strength and conviction is directly thanks to the loss of my first baby. She was Finley's sister.

I know my first baby would have been a girl because I was blessed to have an incredible daytime dream in which I saw her clearly. It was June 2008, a few months after the miscarriage. I was on my own in a forest, setting up a lean-to tent. I had just made a comfy bed of ferns and stood back to take in the stunning rays of sunlight as they cut through the treetops. Out of the corner of my eye, I saw a little girl lying on her back in the bed of ferns, giggling and kicking her legs. I was able to say thank you to her for coming to be with us, and goodbye.

My friend and I also looked at some of the possible reasons I might be feeling so changed within myself. When significant events like this happen, he believes, the shock can affect the personality so deeply that it is destroyed and must be rebuilt. Given my circumstances, it's quite possible that my personality could completely alter. Everything from the way I communicate, the way I relate to people, and what I want for the future – all this could be transformed. I'm intrigued by what my friend is telling me but I'm wondering whether in fact this isn't change as such but instead a return to a more authentic way of being, of expressing what is true at a soul level. At a time before the personality comes to dominate who and what we are.

Perhaps I will shed more and more layers to reveal more and more of the real me. Life is too short to hide me from the world any more. I want my friends and family to know me. I want to be one me all the time, not a different person depending on what I worry people will think. What is there to be frightened of any more? The people that matter the most to me saw me on the worst day of my life, when I was completely unable to hide away. I was totally exposed. That day, the day we buried Finley, my focus was exclusively on what mattered to me and nothing else – myself, Baz and Finley. Nothing else was possible. And that was real. No hiding. It was the worst day of my life and all people could see was strength and dignity. All they could see was love.

At the grave, I hung up a little photo of Finley in a frame that says Shhh baby sleeping. There were other visitors at the cemetery. Imogen's parents were there and another little boy – Joe – had company too. The soil at the bottom of Finley's grave is dropping even more now. Imogen's grave has grass on top and I wonder whether it will drop too and if so how they'll top it up. Imogen's parents have put a black plastic fence around her grave, two black vases for flowers and a little musical box. After Baz left, I sat on a tree stump for a while listening to the wind chimes playing softly. I was the last person in the graveyard once Imogen's parents had left, so I wound up the music box for Imogen and left it tinkling away as I set off for home.

On my way back, I noticed a park near the graveyard. When we have another baby, we'll bring her to see her brother and play in the park. This sets me off on another train of thought. I've been wondering if the Winnie-the-Pooh statue is hollow: if it is, I could place the pregnancy test kit I used when I was pregnant with Finley's sister into it. That way I will feel that I am visiting them both, and that they are together. The test kit is the only memento I have from that pregnancy. There's not even a scan photo. I would've had one if the baby had grown enough for us to see her on the screen. But when we had the scan, we discovered she didn't have a heartbeat.

I got a call from Shirley, the health visitor who runs the baby loss support group. The group meets once a month for two hours in the evening. At the moment, it's women only, but I don't think Baz would be interested anyway. Apparently the mother of the twins buried near Finley goes. Shirley hadn't heard of Imogen, so I might leave a note on her grave to let Imogen's parents know about the group. Shirley will come over in a couple of weeks so that I'll recognise at least one face when I go to the first meeting. It'll be four days after Finley's two-month anniversary.

Day 37

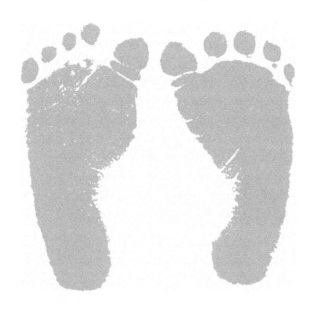

I've realised that I didn't write my note to Finley yesterday. I feel guilty as I hadn't even thought about it. A busy day is no excuse.

I went to see the doctor. I have an eye infection, urine infection and thrush. The heavier bleeding could be due to an internal infection. The doctor has sent for tests, given me eye drops, antibiotics and Canesten. I've got a cold sore too. It certainly shows how well I looked after myself and Finley during pregnancy. How I've let all that go. It was all part of The Gentle Birth Method. I'll definitely follow it next time even though I'll be unlikely to have a natural birth.

I met Sally for lunch. We used to work together and it was great to see her again. We had a good giggle reminiscing about some of the naughty nights out we used to have. We're going to meet again at the end of the month. I've told Baz I want us to visit Wellington one night – there are lots of people who want to catch up with us.

Baz's cousin Robyn has asked for our address. Her gorgeous daughter Ellie has drawn a card for us and a picture for Finley, and wants to send it. Ellie has told all the kids in her class about her cousin who's gone to play with the angels. Children have such a refreshing outlook. They accept what is. If you tell a child that Finley has gone to play with the angels in heaven, then the child will believe you. A child won't apply logic, or start arguing with you or hope to disprove anything. She'll just use her imagination. And what a child can imagine, she can believe. That's freedom.

I've put Finley's photos and videos onto disks and sent one each to Beverly and Liz. I've included a card each too. Congratulations on being Grandparents is printed on the front, and inside I've written Sorry he was not here for longer. I'd seen the same thing in a card Mum's friend Anne had given her, and it touched me.

I've sent Ed and Amie an engagement card, hoping it breaks the awkwardness before my niece is born in October. Our struggles don't change the fact that I want to be the exact same aunty I would have been had we not lost Finley. I need to believe that we will have another baby in our arms soon, and that they will play together just as I'd imagined. It's just that our baby will be the younger one - bossed about by my niece, and protected by my nephew. It's not how we pictured things, but it's okay.

Day 38

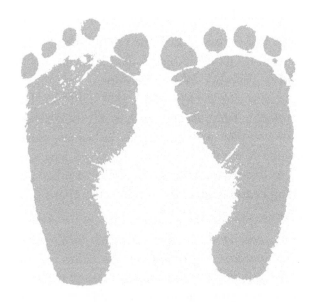

It's 9th September 2009. It's meant to be a special day with magical significance. I'm in Finley's bedroom, it's 9 p.m. and I'm listening to the songs from the funeral.

I walked to Finley's grave in the beautiful sunshine earlier. I was delighted to have managed the two mile round trip there and back. A pleasant walk, it took me past rows of three-storey Victorian houses, with well-tended gardens. I was carrying a very special teddy bear. When I'd woken up this morning, I'd had a clear feeling I should be taking this particular bear to the cemetery with me. We received him in a kit from a charity in the US called A Small Victory. They send the kits to help support people who've suffered miscarriage or baby loss and we'd first contacted them after the miscarriage. Included in the pack is an information brochure, a little birth certificate, a silver heart charm (which Baz now wears on his necklace), and this teddy bear.

I opened the kit to find I'd actually stashed away in it the five pregnancy test sticks I'd used to convince us I was pregnant the first time. Yes, there were five of them! We simply hadn't been able to believe our eyes when we saw the first one was positive. Alongside the test sticks was a tiny pair of white bootees. Wow, as I remembered it, I hadn't bought anything at all for my baby. I must've put them away at the time and never looked in there again. Such a shame. It just doesn't seem enough now that I think of everything I've put together in Finley's memory box. Perhaps I'll make a memory box for his sister too, and keep it alongside Finley's.

So, I took the little brown teddy bear and one of the pregnancy test kits with me to the cemetery. From the side of the road, I picked flowers for my little girl – we've never once given her any. On top of that, I had my journal with me. Just to see if I'd feel able to write a poem while I was at Finley's graveside. A friend had suggested it, just a bit of doodling and a few silly poems. Why not? What if it's actually possible to discover my own sense of fun in the midst of this grief? If I can choose acceptance over denial, and gratitude over anger, why can't I opt for fun over sadness?

Once at the grave, I put down the teddy bear for my little girl in front of Finley's bear. It looks as if they're cuddling each other now. On top of her bear, I laid the freshly picked flowers. Feeling silly now, I buried the pregnancy test kit too. That very second, the wind blew and the wind chimes rang out. I nodded, smiling, and began tending to the grave, watering the flowers, and taking the heads off the lilies the slugs had got to. Clearly slugs don't have much of a taste for chrysanthemums, since they seem to last for ages. I found myself watering the flowers on the other graves too. I like them all to last. So I got a good look around. Imogen's grave now has pink stones on it. Fantastic, if a little lurid! I'll bet they make people grin. There's also a large, colourful grave for a girl called Fiona. It's covered from top to bottom in silk flowers, and edged with multicoloured roses. Fiona had visitors today and they leant me their battery-powered strimmer to cut the grass around Finley's grave. I walked barefoot in the grass, and did write a silly little poem. It's not up to my usual standard, but I'm hopeful it's broken the back of my writer's block.

To Finley,

Your daddy says he will come to see you tomorrow to tell you the result of the football. I spoke to Nana on the phone tonight; she cried when she heard what Imogen's parents wrote in the card they left at your grave. It made me cry, too. Nanny Liz said thank you for the photos.

I'm writing this in your bedroom, Gizmo is asleep in your cot, just where your coffin was, and Mitsi is snuggled next to me, making typing very difficult. They do behave differently in your room; I'm sure they can feel you here.

Tania says that the number nine symbolises endings. Perhaps this year is the end of all the hurt and pain, and next time you come back you will choose to stay. I have been listening to the music from your funeral while I write to you; this time, I'm not crying. You would be happy about that. The lyrics are wonderful.

When you were overdue, I spoke to you and asked you to come and join me, saying that it was time to be born now. Perhaps we live in a time and place where you don't want to be. Maybe you knew that I couldn't change the world, and so you decided to change it so that it is ready for you next time round.

My yesterday won't have to be your way, or my way, or the way for our family.

Day 39

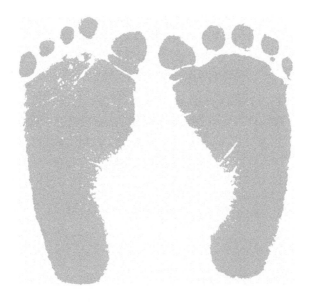

I was up at seven, despite not going to bed before three. I'm tired now after a busy day. Nicola and Terri picked me up at eight thirty for the drive into Bristol. On the way back, I pointed out the cemetery where Finley's grave is.

Terri had eighteen-month-old Percy with her. He's as cute as a button. I sat next to him in the back, playing with his cars. He had me laughing out loud as he yelled an excited Ooh! every time he saw a car or lorry pass by. We accompanied Nicola to hospital for a blood test. She's started her IVF treatment. It's a complicated process and Nicola's finding it hard to stay positive. She doesn't want to get her hopes up or talk about when she's likely to fall pregnant. I wonder if I'd approach it in the same way. If you look at the worst case scenario, you're less likely to be disappointed.

We all needed cheering up, so got together with Nadine for lunch and a bit of shopping. I confided in her some of the more 'out there' things I've been thinking, like my experience with the psychic before I was pregnant, and the Reiki I'd had while pregnant. Nadine's always been interested in clairvoyants, tarot and that kind of thing whereas my naturally analytical mind has until recently made me wary, but things change. Nadine was open to my belief that I'd sensed Finley's soul, even before I was pregnant.

Darren, Hayley and Chloë came over with baby Amber in tow. Darren was really concerned about bringing Amber, but I'm absolutely fine with it now. I was only really upset because Amber cried every time I held her. Of course Baz had no trouble making her smile and laugh. Typical!

To Finley,

Your daddy visited you today and left you a Volkswagen campervan toy and a Spiderman toy. I hope you find a way to say thank you, because these are special to him.

I've been feeling much closer to you today. I've been thinking of you and talking about you, but haven't been sad. I have felt that I am holding you in my arms at times today.

I love you as much as ever and more than before!

Day 40

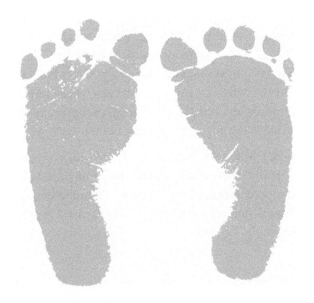

The funeral for my primary school teacher was held today and I didn't go. I didn't want to let go of my good mood. Or have to lift myself up again afterwards. Instead, I went for a long walk along the canal. I fed the ducks and gathered blackberries, things I had loved as a child. I couldn't reach the high branches then, and now that I'm a big girl I still can't get hold of the fattest blackberries. Hilarious.

Taking a moment to be still and enjoy the sunshine, I turned round and caught sight of two exquisite cygnets in the water and a brightly coloured dragonfly close by. It really feels good to immerse myself in the natural world. It's incredibly healing. Things slow down and I'm reminded of the moment I'm in right now. Reminded to enjoy the moment I'm in right here and right now. To stop thinking about the past or worrying about the future,

Finley's collection now totals four hundred and twenty pounds. A work colleague came by with the money she'd collected as well as some more cards. She's invited us to the Christmas Ball. It feels strange to plan so far in advance and yet at the same time good to be making arrangements. Life will move on.

I didn't visit Finley, but bought new flowers to take to him tomorrow.

To Finley,

You would have enjoyed my walk today along the canal to feed the ducks. The sun was shining and it was beautiful. I like to think you joined me. See you tomorrow. Night night, little angel boy.

Day 41

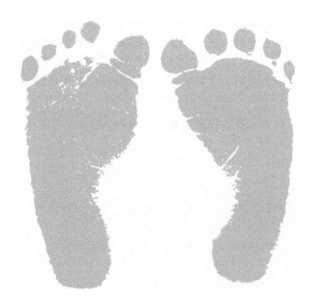

I've felt happy and bouncy all day. The weather is warm and sunny. We took the carnations to Finley but didn't stay long. The soil hasn't been topped up yet. I took my camera with me on my canal walk but didn't see the swans this time. A family with young children paddled by in an open canoe. It reminded me how much Baz and I had enjoyed ourselves canoeing. I'd love to do it again as a family one day. I can just picture us choosing a shady, isolated spot to stop off and have a picnic.

Baz surprised me and walked down to meet me at the canal. I'd already filled up my two pots with blackberries, so he was too late to help me get the juiciest ones from the top branches. We're off to Dartmoor tomorrow for Joanne and Duncan's wedding at the Broken River Hotel. I'm actually looking forward to it, especially the posh room we've booked with four-poster bed and Jacuzzi bath.

To Finley,

I wish you were coming with us tomorrow to share the special hotel. I will think of you often so it will feel as if you are there.

Day 42

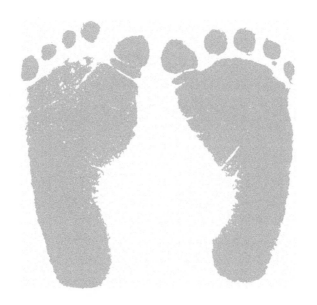

The wedding was the first family occasion we've been to since Finley and it hit us both hard. Our baby is not here. There is someone missing. When we arrived at the hotel, I opened the wardrobe door to hang up our clothes, and there, to my horror, was the travel cot we'd ordered back before Finley was born. The hotel staff hadn't removed it as we'd asked. What a shock.

In her speech, Joanne talked about Finley. We all cried, but it was so much better having her acknowledge the elephant in the room than not. Next to the wedding cake, Joanne had placed a collection pot, Finley's photograph and a candle. So he could join in on her special day. By the end of the day, people had donated a total of one hundred and twenty pounds. I kept moving the photo around to make sure Finley could see all the different parts of the room. Then, in the wedding guest book, I left a special message from him.

Bernie, Joanne's godson, was born too soon. His mum was at the wedding and I was glad to get the chance at last to meet her. She reassured me that things do get better. In fact, she's pregnant again now.

At one point in the afternoon, I was sitting near the bar when a woman promptly sat down next to me and started to feed her baby. Anything else but this I could have managed. But there's something so special about a woman feeding her baby. It's absolutely beautiful. Nurturing and peaceful. There they were in a room full of people, yet totally – exclusively – focused on one another. I would give anything to have that. I rushed out of the room in tears. Beverley saw me and chased after me. By the time she found me, she was weeping too.

I was woken in the middle of the night by a thought that repeated itself over and over in my mind: we are loved and protected. At the same time, I could see a pink light surrounding the two of us as we lay there in bed. I realised I'd felt this before. Just after we first left the hospital, I'd woken up time and again with this same pink light encircling us. And the phrase – I am in love – running over repeatedly in my mind. I am in love. I know this to mean I am immersed in and surrounded by love.

Day 43

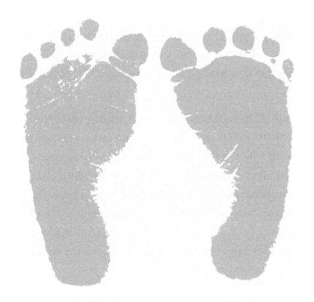

We left the hotel after a delicious breakfast. But we were late and I was in trouble, since I hadn't been able to drag myself out of the Jacuzzi in time. I realised on the way home that I'd left my bracelet at the hotel. The one Nadine gave me at Finley's funeral. I hope I get it back.

We stopped on the way home to take photos of the wild ponies on Dartmoor. We were able to get right up close to them and their foals, so the photos were pretty spectacular.

Day 44

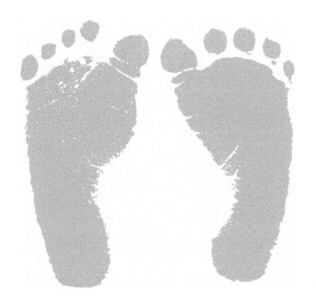

The doctor has prescribed me more antibiotics. If only my body would get back to normal. At least I'm allowed to drive now, and go swimming, which I'm really looking forward to. It will be strange learning to swim again without a bump. When you're heavily pregnant and swim on your belly, you start to sink. But if you swim on your back, the bump makes you roll over! The strangest sensation of all is when you're swimming and the baby moves inside you.

I'd planned to go back to Bumps and Beyond after Finley was born. It's a pre and postnatal water aerobics class. I can't see how I can do it now as I'd have to explain the whole thing to all the girls I knew there. It wouldn't be fair on them. I wouldn't want them to feel awkward, or worry that the same thing might happen to them. So I'll leave it until I'm pregnant again.

My close work colleague visited. She's concerned that I haven't been eating and drinking enough, and she's heard I've been ill. I think she may be worried I'm becoming depressed. I'm not. I'm even eating a little better now. Those first few weeks, I was in shock. I had no appetite at all. But that's changing, and I actually feel hungry these days. The eating plan has helped too, even though I'm still tending to eat at unusual times.

I've told her we'll come to the Christmas Ball. It's being held at a really posh school, so we'll have the chance to dress up. I still get that feeling of being pulled two ways emotionally when we talk about Christmas: I'm excited to be looking forward to something but it's a real wrench to acknowledge that life is moving on. We're actually hoping to stay with Baz's cousin in Germany in December.

So I've said I'll probably come back to work after Christmas. It's still too soon right now and I don't even want to go into the office yet. I'd like to see my team, but not everyone else. I don't want to have to answer too many questions right now. Still, it's interesting to be told that people are worrying about me. Interesting to notice how often I'm feeling good. Especially when expectations are the opposite.

I'm starting to realise how significant this is. So I've been reflecting on the grief cycle and where I am in it. If I am in it.

You're expected to pass through all sorts of stages. If I have chosen to accept that Finley died, where exactly do I fit into the cycle? I'm not in a state of denial or resistance but one of acceptance. I've done many things to allow this to take place. It's totally different to what I experienced after the miscarriage last year. Then, I spent a lot of time trying to get through my pain by thinking about the pregnancy as if it had been postponed and trying to get pregnant again as soon as possible. That was denial. I had no choice eventually but to accept the reality of what had happened. But that didn't start until I held Jade's baby Harvey. I cried then, seeing the miscarriage for what it was for the very first time: the loss of my baby. I wanted to stop trying for a baby then and told Baz as much. Each month when my period arrived had been like having the miscarriage all over again. Of course, that was when I got pregnant with Finley.

This time I understand that I have helped myself accept that Finley is dead. At first, when I was in hospital with him, I needed to care for him, to mother him, as much as I could. I needed to acknowledge my maternal feelings and allow them to be expressed. Of course, very obvious things were missing. I couldn't feel, hear or see Finley breathing. I couldn't feed him. His nappy was not wet even though we changed it. He didn't have that new baby smell. His fingers didn't close around mine as I held his hand. None of these things took place as they would have done had he been alive. I knew my baby was dead. But I had to care for him as though he were alive. It was the first stage of the process. The second stage was to see Finley's body in the coffin, and to bring him home in it. This time we didn't hold him. We knew he was dead. We knew that what had made him Finley had left that body.

So, what does it mean to say I have chosen to accept that Finley died? It means I feel profound gratitude for all the gifts he has left. It means I am not angry. It means that while I still feel sadness from time to time, the sadness is alright. It's okay to feel sad. All kinds of things can set me off, bring tears to my eyes. And that is fine. It is as it is.

I suspect that acceptance also means I am choosing for myself the way that I grieve. That it's actually possible to choose the way you grieve. Just as it feels possible for this tragic thing to be a positive experience. It feels possible that there is another way through this. I mean, I'm learning so much, so many new and wonderful things. And I'm questioning everything I once thought to be true. All the beliefs that have held me back before no longer exist. In fact, these 'beliefs', these things we think are so concrete, are actually flexible! I can change them. So, if nothing is the way I once believed, then the time is truly right for me to create the future I want. I can build new beliefs that fit with my new experience of life. What happens if I choose to create new beliefs that will only help and not hinder me? If I can change my beliefs, what will I choose? What will I be; what will I do? What am I truly capable of in this life?

To Finley,

Your daddy and I had a lovely time at the weekend. We are enjoying our marriage and our time together – I hope you can see it.

I saw so many white feathers at the weekend, I was thinking of you a lot. I will ignore the fact that there were four white geese outside the hotel creating all the feathers!

I popped in to see you quickly this morning. I will visit for longer another day. Love you lots and lots baby.

Day 45

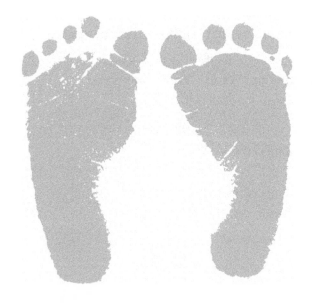

Baz's first day back at work. His boss has been very understanding. Baz has just discovered that one of his workmates has twin boys buried a few graves down from Finley. They died at twenty-two weeks.

I enjoyed my first day alone. Baz called at nine-thirty and I couldn't get back to sleep so it gave me good reason to get up. I had an orange, pineapple and blackberry juice. The spiritualist church nearby offers a drop-in healing session on a Wednesday, so, despite not knowing what to expect, I decided to turn up. A kind man called Ray was on duty. He put me at ease quickly. I felt heat through his hands and it really alleviated the strain in my neck. We also worked on the area around my scars which he recommended I can do by myself any time. Ray actually helped me connect again with the spirits the psychic had revealed to me last year. I didn't mention a thing about them to Ray until after the session was over.

Then I explained all about Finley. Ray was thankful for it as it helped him feel more able to offer his compassion and share his knowledge. I also confided in him some of the things I've learnt since Finley was born. That I know Finley visited us to do a job, that all kinds of healing have taken place as a result. Ray said he saw Finley with two spirits in white. He called them the white brotherhood. They were there to help guide Finley's soul and teach him how to communicate. The communication between Finley and me will improve, Ray said, the more Finley learns. This reassures me. Although I remain somewhat sceptical, it is sweet to think that Finley may be able to speak to me in the future.

I've joined the library. I've always enjoyed reading and have already ordered several books about baby loss.

To Finley,

I've had an amazing day today: I've thought about you often. I am happy and excited and learning a lot, and this is because of what happened to you.

I love you so much, and am grateful to you every day, my baby boy. Enjoy being with the angels.

Day 46

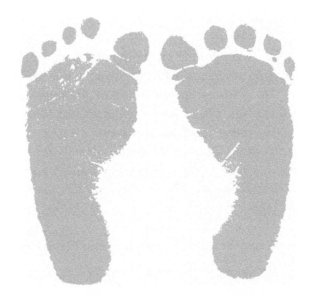

I went swimming for the first time since Finley was born and had to walk to Baz's work to collect the car. As I'd expected, going swimming without my bump was disconcerting. Everything I did reminded me of what it was like before. When I had a shower, I saw my reflection in the same mirror where I used to check out the differences in my bump every week. In the changing rooms, I caught sight of the same playpen that I used to look at, thinking, I'll be able to put my baby in there soon. It's definitely easier to swim without a bump though, since I don't feel half as heavy in the water. I miss being pregnant.

Only forty-two days after leaving hospital, and I've been brave enough to unpack one of my bags. I've decided to keep some of the things I'd prepared for my labour in a box ready for next time. Because there will be a next time. It's difficult to describe the emotions I felt unpacking all those baby clothes and nappies. It wasn't sadness as such but the sense that I'm missing out. A sense of how much I'm missing out on. There were all the clothes I'll never dress Finley in, the nappies I'll never change for him. I wish things were different. Is there really anything wrong with feeling this? I know I can't change anything, that we can't go back, and that Finley won't be in our future in the way we'd hoped and planned. I still can't help but wish things were different.

To Finley,

I miss you so much. I have a room full of clothes that you will never wear. I have a shelf full of books you'll never read. I have a pushchair that I will not push you in. I have an armful of cuddles that you will not feel again, and a zillion kisses that I can only blow towards you. I wish you were here.

Day 47

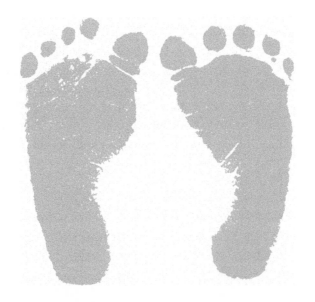

I slept so well that I didn't get up until eleven even after an early night. Baz made it to work, so the early night must have done him good too. I walked over to Katy's for a cup of tea. On the way back, I picked more blackberries by the canal. I wish I'd taken my camera, as there were some divine little baby moorhens sitting on the reeds. It's important to be out and about in the natural world like this. Not just because it relaxes me. But also because it helps bring me more fully into the present moment. Stops me replaying the past or getting anxious about the future. Nature definitely works some kind of healing magic on me.

It was good to see Katy. We talked about the healing session at the spiritualist church and she told me what to expect next time. There'll be clairvoyant readings. I'm going with an open mind and am looking forward to meeting others. Katy says she was one of the youngest people there. Somehow I'd thought it would be full of younger people. You expect them to be more open-minded.

I got the chance to cuddle Danni's baby Isabelle. She's such a smiley baby, it was wonderful to hug her and play with her. Mum called to tell me that my brother Stephen's girlfriend Denise has been to hospital for a scan as they were worried the baby wasn't growing. He's due in just over two weeks. He's fine, already weighing six pounds. The hospital offered to induce Denise because of her Braxton Hicks contractions. They were both shocked, but want to wait until full term. Denise will have another scan before then just to stay sure the baby is still growing.

Stephen has asked Mum if Baz and I have any smaller newborn baby clothes since they think the stuff they've bought might be too big now. I feel okay about this, and I'll put an M on them, so we can have them back when we have our baby.

To Finley,

I have learnt that I can miss you without being sad. I am bound to miss you, I love you and you are not here. I can miss you, and miss the experience of being pregnant with you, but it does not have to make me miserable. I think you'd like that. I wish things were different, even while I accept the way they are.

Day 48

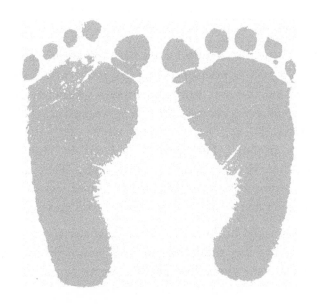

An evening of clairvoyance with Katy at the spiritualist church. I hadn't been sure what to expect and started out pretty sceptical given the vague and generalised messages the medium gave out. Most of what he said to others could easily have applied to me and my situation. However, all of a sudden, I sensed that the medium was about to approach me. He walked straight over and looked me directly in the eyes. Pins and needles shot down my right side. He told me that a lady was standing near me, a grandmotherly presence. That things had been difficult for me for some time now. He could sense an opportunity for me – November would be an important time. It all sounded vaguely relevant, but pretty broad and not very persuasive. He spoke again: she is saying that she wants to fatten you up because you have lost weight. Then he came up with something that really did get my attention. He said he was being given a cheese and onion sandwich. Now, cheese and onion sandwiches are honestly my favourite and I had literally only just eaten one before I came out. I sat there racking my brains trying to remember if perhaps I'd spoken to the medium earlier and he could have smelt the onion on my breath. I hadn't.

To Finley,

I find it very comforting to think that you may still be able to see me and that one day you might be able to give us a message. I like to think that you can guide me and your daddy through the important decisions we need to make.

I know you are a very old soul, and very wise. I am honoured that you chose us as your parents. I love you always my baby boy.

Day 49

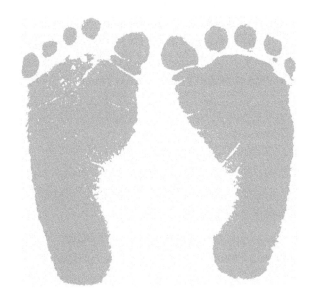

Daddy Baz found the strimmer and cut down the jungle on the front drive. It had been threatening to overwhelm the whole house. It's seven weeks since Finley was born. Seven weeks today. I can't believe it. It feels like a whole lifetime has passed in those seven weeks. And yet it could have been just a minute ago I first saw his face.

I've found Facebook really useful all this time. Posting status updates has meant that people haven't had to contact us every second to see how we are. Friends and family can read about us online and keep up to date that way. On days I've posted I'm having a bad time, or similar, we've had heaps of calls. Today was the first time our friend Clive, who lives nearby, has been to see us since Finley. He's wanted to give us the time and space we need. And he's been keeping up with us on Facebook just to make sure the time is right.

I went to the spiritualist church alone tonight since Katy wasn't feeling well. There was a fairly normal church service. We sang the same hymns as you would at any other church, and there was an address and a reading from the bible. I don't much like that part of it; I don't think church is for me. I enjoy prayer, and the fact the prayers talk about sending healing and light to people in need. But I'm more interested in the spiritualist readings. That's what I came for tonight.

The guest speaker gave out messages after the service. One was for me. There was an elderly lady, he said. At first I thought it could be Nana, like last night. But no, this woman had died around the time I was born. She had only known me when I was a babe in arms. I thought it could have been Dad's mum, but she died when I was seven. The speaker continued, saying that I'd turned a corner. According to this elderly lady, I wouldn't simply be handed an answer to my little problem (and he emphasised the word little). In finding that answer, I'd also learn to stand on my own two feet. Go in good cheer, the lady said. But the medium also had a warning for me. Very shortly, I would notice someone very close to me doing something, speaking or acting in a manner that was totally out of character. I wonder what this could be! Still, I can't understand why Finley doesn't send me a message. I would love so much to hear from him.

When I got home, I called Mum. She told me that her Gran had died when I was a baby, and had only met me a couple of times when I was tiny.

To Finley,

I wonder if you are the little problem the speaker was referring to? Or maybe he was talking about my wish to have a baby in general? I wonder whether you will come to visit with a message when I see Vernon for the reading? I would like so much to hear from you again. Mummy and Daddy love you lots and lots – a zillion times more than infinity.

Day 50

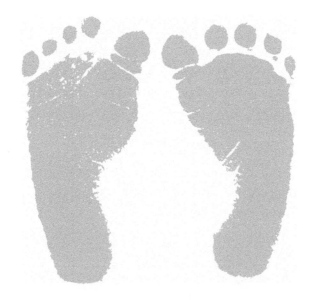

I've been cheerful and in a cheeky mood all day long. I'm rebuilding my whole belief system, you know! I've been discussing it on the phone with a good friend of mine. Other people are really interested in these lessons I'm learning, and that surprises me. The fact is, my experiences have completely removed my foundations from under me. I have no choice but to rebuild from scratch. On a daily basis, no experience I'm having corresponds with anything I've ever believed to be true. I have to work fast to keep up with all these lessons I need to learn.

For a start, I haven't been feeling the emotions normally associated with grieving. I suppose it worries me a bit. But I just don't feel sad, angry, resentful, or in denial. Sure, I may have moments where I feel these things. But they are fleeting. There's a whole host of things I do to keep such moments brief. If I can simply be in the moment, then the emotions just aren't harmful. I can have tears rolling down my face, and not actually be in pain. Also, if I accept that I am feeling a difficult emotion, such as sadness, then it doesn't hurt. And, as soon as I recognise the sadness, I find ways to change it. These are similar to the strategies I've been teaching others for a long time. Like teaching distraction techniques to people suffering from anxiety.

I've given all this a good deal of thought. When I play a relaxation CD, listen to music, go for a walk, read a book, swim or write, I am immersing myself in the present moment. I am in the here and now. Attending to what is right here before me. Alerting my senses. I'm not losing myself in thought about what has been, what might have been or could come to be.

In one sense, these activities are a distraction from thoughts that make me sad; but they are also more than a distraction. They are a way of removing the habits of thought from an experience. Removing the judgements that cause us to suffer. They offer a way of seeing through the veil of fearful thinking and into the light of presence. They are helping me just to be. To exist peacefully in the here and now, in the present moment.

I can feel very strongly a part of me, deep within, that is peaceful and content even when my mind is racing. This I call my inner person. If I can connect with this part of myself, with this peace and calm, this stillness within, then my mind is free. Free to have the thoughts without those thoughts becoming harmful to me. For example, I can have the thought that Finley was born seven weeks ago. Now the thought itself can conjure up many possible meanings, interpretations or judgements. It could bring with it feelings of sadness, resentment, bitterness or anger. Or it could bring relief, happiness or joy. The thought – Finley was born seven weeks ago – doesn't actually have a fixed value attached to it. It's just a thought. It's not necessarily a sad thought. Only once I start to make judgements about it does the thought become either a painful or a joyful thought. Judgements like it shouldn't be this way. Or I don't deserve this.

Look at it this way. If someone with no knowledge of my story were to read the words exactly as I have written them – Finley was born seven weeks ago – that person might be more likely to read in them happiness, joy, wonder, or pride, than sadness or pain. After all, a child was born, right? This is important. It's got to be possible to detach your thoughts from the strong emotional effects they appear to evoke. And there's another thing. I seem to talk about the fact that Finley was born. When did I stop referring to the day when Finley died? What a world of difference between the two versions of the story I choose to tell myself. What a world of difference between the way I feel as a result.

So, this much is clear. When my inside person is peaceful and relaxed, the thoughts have no emotion attached to them. They are thoughts and are noted for their value, but they do no harm. It's a subtle difference. Not so long ago, any such thought would've made me miserable instantly. But now there's something different going on. I'm still processing all this of course. Still working it out. In some ways it's really very clear. In others, I worry it won't make sense to read. But look, if I'm thinking about the past or planning for the future, rather than being in the present, then I feel the negative feelings. I actually feel them. In a way, even this goes against what I'm trying to say here. I mean, the term negative feelings itself implies a judgement. Maybe I'll do a Prince (remember how he dropped the name Prince and became the artist formerly known as Prince?). Then I can talk about the feelings formerly considered to be negative!

Anyway, I've got to get to the bottom of this. So let's say I'm sitting here thinking about the past. Thinking about the miscarriage. In that case, if I have the thought Finley was born seven weeks ago, I immediately fall into a spiral of despair, with thoughts such as it's so unfair, why have I lost a second baby, why did this happen to me again? I'm making a judgement about what's happening now and I'm looking to the past as evidence to back up my story. Something's happening to me. I don't deserve it. It's not fair. All that kind of thing. I'm making all sorts of inferences about the present moment based on judgements I've made about what's past. Now, because of this, because I'm sitting there in the past, this string of thoughts feels painful. It hurts me and makes me feel sad or angry. But when I connect with my inner person, with that sense of calm and peace within, I simply can't feel those emotions any more. My inner person values the thought for what it is – a statement marking the time that has passed since Finley was born. It's as simple as that.

Shirley the health visitor didn't seem to believe me when I told her I was feeling good. She'd come over to introduce herself before I go to the baby loss support group. She wanted to know how we're coping. A lovely lady, but like everyone, it's somehow easier for her to hear me say I feel terrible or it's so awful. People just don't seem to get it if I say I'm okay. So I've given up.

Shirley tells me there's around six to eight people who go to the group regularly, mums from all different circumstances. She kept calling the people that go along mums. I wanted to say to her I won't fit in, I'm not a mum, I have no children. She said that some people have been going to the group for years. I'm not sure how healthy that can be, but when I questioned it, Shirley said that although you might expect the group to be a sad place, for the mums it's a real tonic. Women have made lasting friendships there and some weeks no one even mentions babies at all. This has raised some interesting questions for me. I think I'd prefer a more structured group. I wonder why the group has no resources? It's clearly a much needed service. I want to look into it more.

Since Baz is back at work, I thought I'd cook tea. I'm not sure how, but it's clearly possible to burn food in the oven while at the same time under-cooking rice on the hob! I'm such a terrible wife.

Day 51

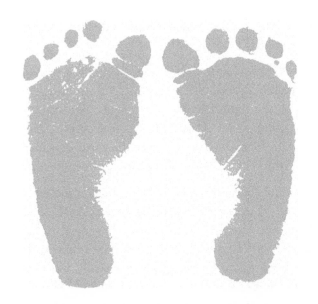

I've been keeping myself busy deleting old emails. I ran across one I'd sent to a woman who runs a website about communication with babies before birth. I'd written to her after we lost our first baby, when I'd just got pregnant with Finley. I'm intrigued to discover that at such an early stage in the pregnancy I was already starting to explore my beliefs about the connection I was to experience so deeply later on.

I was up late last night writing and talking to a friend, so I'm tired. At least it meant Baz got some sleep. It's harder to stay in a positive frame of mind when we're both tired. You really can't overestimate the importance of good nutrition, and getting good quality and enough sleep. Caring for my body is vital if I'm going to carry on supporting my mental and emotional state. I've noticed this in the past. If I'm low or stressed out it goes hand in hand with letting my physical health slide out of control. This has meant I've remained in emotional pain for a long time.

Over at Katy's, Jacqui cut my hair. There's something wonderful about looking and feeling good. It helps put a value on you and on your life. It's not something I've placed a great deal of importance on in the past. I've never really taken all that much care of my appearance. But now I realise there's really something to be said for it. It's not about vanity. Nothing like that. It's about feeling good. And I like feeling good. I want to care for myself and feel good all the time. Right now, I'm blessed to have the time and space to explore what helps me feel good. It's just common-sense stuff this. There's no secret to it.

A few weeks back, having my hair cut could easily have upset me. I'd have seen it as another sign of life moving on and so moving away from Finley. Now I'm excited at how life has been, and how our life will be. I'm looking forward to tomorrow. I have some books to collect from the library, and I'll be off to the spiritualist church for a meditation session and the healing drop-in.

To Finley,

I spoke to Alex last night. She said she feels as if she knows you.

I told her I've realised that I can bring you alive through writing. Anything is possible – in life and in fiction.

When our kitten Squidgy died, I wanted to write a series of children's storybooks about Squidgy's adventures. Now Squidgy has an owner to create havoc together with him.

Perhaps through my writing I will be able to see you eating worms in the garden, squirting the cats with the hose pipe, playing in the park, having your first day at school, passing your exams, having your driving test, getting married.

I love you more than ever, baby boy.

Day 52

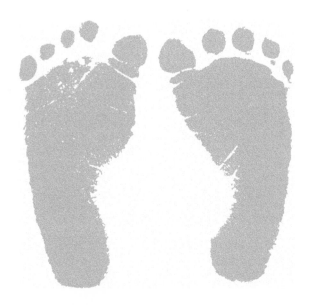

I've been a bit less upbeat today. Perhaps because I'm eating wheat again, maybe because of this infection, or the side effects of the antibiotics. Or it could just be one of those days. I'll refrain from labelling it either way. It's neither good nor bad. It's just a day.

I was a bit nervous at first at the spiritualist church meditation session. But once Ray had explained that he was going to lead us in a guided visualisation, I was pretty comfortable. I've been teaching guided visualisation myself for years now. Ray explained that he'd take us to an imaginary place and leave us there in the silence for five minutes at first, then later for ten. I was worried the meditation would be too long at that rate. But I had no trouble at all once we got going. I was surprised to find, when Ray brought us back to the room, that a whole thirty-five minutes had passed. My level of relaxation had deepened at each stage. And I discovered that focusing on my breathing and counting as I went was a great way to remain in that meditative space. I find it easier to relax when someone's talking. Otherwise my thoughts tend to float around in the silence and that distracts me. Still, that's the nature of meditation. Thoughts are given the opportunity to surface. I wonder if meditation is the best space in which to explore the thoughts or whether I should just watch them come up?

The guided visualisation involved decorating a room in any way we wanted. I designed a turquoise room with butterflies fluttering about in it. I didn't so much see it as an image in my mind's eye but more as if I was reading it out loud or telling a story to myself and feeling the emotions. I added some pictures to my room and when I included a photo of Finley it changed into a swinging cot. As I watched it swing, I felt Finley just behind me, out a little to the left. Something started glowing there at the precise moment Ray started talking about a golden healing light coming through a skylight in the room, into the top of our head. I felt the light as a beam of energy, and then was able to imagine it flowing down through me. It was the same feeling I'd experienced during Reiki, when my awareness moved from the top of my head, down and out of my body. I'm almost certain I'm still connecting with Finley at times like this. Unless it's a memory, or a deeply held wish.

When I got home, Jodie had sent me some beautiful music via Facebook. The music made me cry and I ended up feeling a bit flat. So, at a friend's suggestion, I took a bath with lavender oil and sea salt while listening to uplifting music. It worked and my mood improved.

At the church, a woman had handed me a large, round orange dahlia. So I took it to Finley and laid it on his grave. Like a little piece of sunshine. The grave next to Finley's had been tidied up. Now there's only a few plants recently laid in the bare soil. All the toys have been placed in a plastic carrier bag. I wonder if the cemetery staff tidied it up. I also noticed that Imogen's grave no longer has pink stones on it.

I picked up a bag full of cute little girl's clothes from Freecycle to give to Ed. I got a big bunch of toys too, and, as I was dividing them up to share between our niece and nephew (both expected soon), Baz asked for one. Then another. I wondered why and must have looked puzzled. He said keep that one for our baby, and this one's for Finley. Finley will always will be included.

To Finley,

I love you so much. I never imagined it was possible to love anything this much. I feel like I will burst, I am so full up with this love.

I can see you everywhere, in everything. Yesterday another white feather blew right across in front of me as I was walking along the road. Had I been in the cemetery, I wouldn't have been half as surprised. That place is full of white feathers. However, I like to think it was you reminding me you're there.

I thought of you today when I saw the big sunshiney flower. I hope it makes you smile too. We will come to see you soon and bring the pressies with us.

Day 53

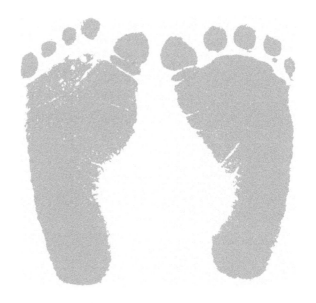

I'm busy but exhausted. I may have overestimated how much I can take on. I'm losing my patience with people, and struggle to concentrate long enough for good conversation.

I went to visit Stephen and Denise. Their baby is due soon. They were happy with the toys, books and clothes I gave them. Denise has a small, football-shaped bump. I have been broody, trying to get pregnant, or pregnant for so long that I feel conditioned to be excited about anything baby-related. No matter how I feel, the excitement's still there. So I cooed over the nursery. It's strange to see my younger brother excited about being a dad. In my mind's eye he's still the little curly-haired lad who demanded his hair be cut because people thought he was a girl, who used to run around naked in front of my friends. He's all grown up now.

My mood stayed high for a good while, even when I spoke about Finley. I compared how big Finley was with how tiny their baby will be. Denise will be having a scan tomorrow and might be induced if he hasn't grown since the last one. So I could be an aunty very soon. While part of me is excited about it, another part is gutted not to be a mum. It's just the way it is and I accept it.

I had no patience in the swimming pool afterwards. What a challenge. I swam fifteen lengths in just twenty minutes but then got out because other people were going too slowly. I was incensed that the lifeguard wouldn't let me swim in the fast lane but wouldn't move the slow people from the slow lane either.

I visited Chloë and baby Honey; Hayley and baby Amber were there too. I enjoyed a long cuddle with Honey who laughed and was then sick on me twice. Charming. It gets easier each time I'm with someone's baby, though it's tough as I see what I'm missing.

The doctor recommended that Baz doesn't drive the forklift as his concentration is affected by his grief. He received an invitation to the children's Christmas party at work and it upset him so much he was sent home. I wish I could have been at home with him.

When I did get home, we had to take the cat to the vet. Goodness, I've been a model of activity. So much in so little time. I suspect I need to take a break during the day specially for myself. I should sit in the park or something. Now I'm stressing about tomorrow's list, which includes an appointment with a counsellor.

Day 54

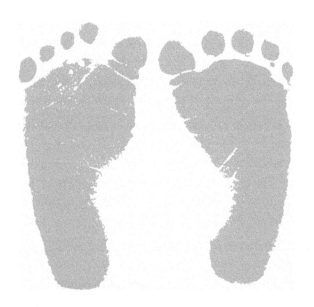

I should learn never to pre-judge. There I was worrying about today and it turned out to be so tranquil. No need to worry at all. I'm not sure this counsellor has ever had a client quite like me. I made it clear that I'm well aware of the grief cycle and the things I should be doing and feeling. Then I insisted she take care of the language she uses: she told me I would have good and bad days and I do not find this helpful at all. You'd think a counsellor would know about self-fulfilling prophecy! If she tells me I'll be likely to have bad days, then I'll be likely to have bad days.

Anyway, the counsellor asked me some initial questions to get a handle on how I'm doing. The idea was to repeat the questions at the end of the session to evaluate my progress. I answered the questionnaire honestly. It was interesting to rate my moods and to acknowledge how good I've been feeling this last week. I told her I had concerns that this positive feeling was false. A kind of mask. But I know this is a fear. Not the truth at all. Then, when I talked to her about my experiences of Being in the present moment, I discovered that psychotherapists have a term for it. It's known as mindfulness.

The counsellor asked if I would like to see her again. I think I would. So we've arranged an appointment for next week. I honestly have no idea how I'm going to deal with the next few months. What with the babies about to be born to close friends and family, Christmas on the way, and the results from Finley's post-mortem due any time now, it's comforting to know I can get support from the counsellor if I need it. She's offered to meet Baz too, if he'll agree.

Baz wants to think about coming with me. He's been trying to be strong for Finley and for me, but says he's finding it hard to let go. I asked him what he was worried about. He said he fears if he lets go he could have a nervous breakdown. How do I tell him this isn't going to happen? It's only if he keeps his emotions bottled up inside that it could. There's so much support available for him if I can't contain his emotions safely by myself. But no one will help if he doesn't reach out. I wonder if this is another of Finley's gifts. Is he showing us that people will give if only they are asked? Is he showing us how easily kindness comes? That all you have to do is ask? Yes, Finley is showing us that there is another way. Another way through life than pain, suffering or separation. And that this is love.

I find that I want to be surrounded by beautiful things and bright colours. Baz knows it – he's just bought me a bunch of dazzling purple and pink flowers.

To Finley,

You are forever in the front of my mind, my heart and my thoughts. You are in a white feather, a butterfly, the rays of sunshine, the petals of a flower, the clouds in the sky, the breeze through the trees. You are never lost because beauty is everywhere and beauty reminds me of you.

The counsellor asked me today why I said I didn't feel brave enough to go back for Reiki and reflexology with Lynne. I replied that our connection during those sessions had been so special and strong that I'd miss it if I went back. Perhaps in time I'll go back and it'll give me a safe space to remember all you were. Perhaps I will be able to smile at the memory of you. I think I'll try it again when I'm pregnant with your brother or sister.

Day 55

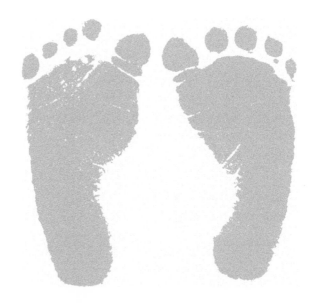

Beverley and Mick invited us to Butlins in Minehead for the day. I took Beverley to Horner Woods for a cup of tea and a cake. There's an old, converted watermill there, now someone's house, fronted by rows of vivid sunflowers. Although I was anxious at first, things went smoothly. I still go quiet when I'm in social situations, finding myself wanting to scream out my baby died! But we were both pretty comfortable with the quieter moments. At Porlock beach, we picked up stones for Finley: one in the shape of a heart, the other a teardrop.

I think I'll be planting my own sunflowers next year. There's something about a sunflower that makes the corners of my mouth curl up.

Day 56

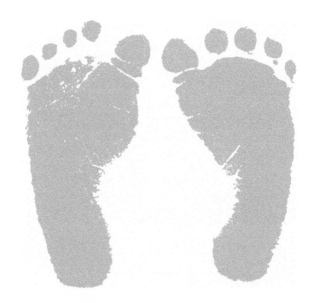

At the spiritualist church, Katy and I saw the medium, Vernon, for a private reading. There were lots of spirits around me, Vernon said. A lady's energy is surrounding me with love. There's also a young energy – a young girl who loves animals. He said that sometimes I feel as if things are going away from me, but that everything happens for a reason. Who's the driver? he asked. So I replied that both Baz and I drive. Vernon could see someone – a spirit? – sitting in the back of a car with their hands over their eyes. I caught Katy's eye and we giggled. Baz drives like a racing-car driver most of the time and I have to hang on for dear life!

Vernon said that Baz can be quite impatient, but also that the spirits are telling me I will not have to go through this again. I'm happy about that; I have been through this twice and that is enough. He said that I've been wondering why this has happened, since other people don't seem to have problems. That I need to focus on the future, as the past has passed. That I must feel the love around me, and start to feel good about myself.

The reading had enough specific points that I found it easy to believe in the spirits around me, looking after my best interests. But what gets me more is the idea that the soul continues after the body dies. That I find comforting.

On the way to collect Baz, I drove past the cemetery, so dropped in to visit Finley. There was a bit of a crowd there and I got to meet them all: Imogen's parents, Cameron and Carter's mum, Joe's mum and Mia's dad. We sat on the grass together chatting and swapping stories. We shared Facebook details, and offered to support each other. Under other circumstances this would have been a pleasant, friendly little gathering. But there was something really tragic about us all being there. With the exception of Mia, all our babies had been lost within two months of each other.

We've arranged to meet up for the International Wave of Light event that's organised as part of International Pregnancy and Baby Loss Awareness Day. We'll meet at the cemetery and, like thousands of others around the globe, light candles for our babies at seven in the evening and leave them to burn for an hour, creating a wave of light around the world. I can only imagine how beautiful this will be. We've agreed to read out a poem too. I'll be lighting a candle for Finley, of course. And for his sister.

Day 57

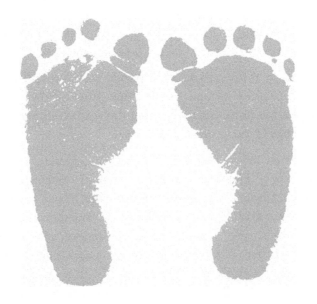

I've been enjoying myself listening to music on You Tube and turning it up LOUD. Songs for Finley. I've been making sure I alternate between sad songs and more uplifting ones to keep my mood buoyant. It really is good to allow myself the time to think of him. There's actually a whole bunch of great little tunes out there written especially about angel babies. Some of them can be downloaded free to use for tributes and on websites.

Beverley and Mick called in on their way back from Minehead. They'd been to see Finley. Now there's a butterfly on his grave, and stones too with love and joy on them. They'd picked up a badge for Finley at Butlins and they pinned it to his teddy bear. I'm delighted because now Finley has had his first holiday. His wind chimes were playing the whole time they were at the grave, Beverley said.

I've been added as a friend on Facebook by lots of people who've also lost babies. People I can speak to who would understand. It's comforting to know they're there. At the same time, I feel blessed to be feeling the way I'm feeling. There's such gratitude in me. There's always sadness too, of course, but it's surrounded with a kind of awareness and clarity. I can easily see how my feelings could become overwhelming. But they're not. They're like signposts towards something new and brilliant.

We've just discovered that we're not entitled to Child Benefit or Child Trust Fund money because Finley didn't take a breath. He was forty-one weeks and five days old and he had a heartbeat all through the labour. But he couldn't hang on long enough to take a breath. Parents of a baby who takes a single breath and then dies would qualify for the benefits. But not us. We could have put the money towards the cost of Finley's headstone. Now we'll have to find another way to save up for it. I met a woman on Facebook who runs a charity in memory of her daughter Megan and wants to raise money to help parents buy headstones for their angel babies. I wonder if she has any ideas.

To Finley,

You will have lots of friends to play with wherever you are. There are so many of you who come to visit for a little while, but do not stay for long.

Your daddy asked me to tell you the football scores. I think he said Plymouth lost 1 – 0 to Liverpool. I am sure there was lots more I was supposed to tell you about penalties and stuff but you know I don't like football.

Did you move the remote control earlier? Your daddy couldn't find it!

Day 58

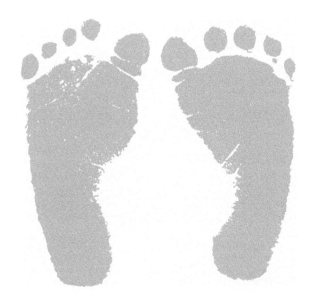

I can't begin to grasp the fact that almost sixty days have passed since Finley was born. It will be his two-month anniversary on Thursday. Time stands still and yet has flown by. Wasn't it just yesterday I was pregnant, waiting impatiently for my due date to arrive?

I am full of energy and exhausted at the same time. After an early start, I'd dozed off by mid-morning. I need to start getting used to the idea of going to work at some point, so I've agreed to meet Nikki for coffee. It'll be a good habit to get into.

I'm thinking about Baz and his Xbox. He needs to send it off for repairs, so I walked into town to collect some bubble wrap. As I was walking, I started thinking this Xbox is much more than just a boys' toy. The Xbox is to Baz what Facebook is to me. A way to connect to people. To feel less alone.

In town, I bought Finley a cute teddy bear snow globe For a Special Baby Boy. I caught a glimpse of a really nice angel calendar too. But I started to think of time rushing by, and of all the firsts I'd miss marking down. First birthday, first Mother's Day, first Father's Day. First anniversary. There's just the one date for Finley really. Just one. My baby was born and died on the same day.

At the grave, we ran into Donna whose little boy Joe is buried at the end of Finley's row. She'd been clearing leaves from the graves and was saying goodbye. We did some maintenance too, getting rid of fallen leaves and cutting the overlong grass. There's still no one to ask about topping up the soil. We want to lay stones and put up a green fence – the Plymouth Argyle club colours. We'll add a badge for Finley too. The fence can go up at the weekend, with Finley's photo frame on it.

I contacted CJ Ballas, the author of Finlay's Garden, a children's book that deals with the death of a baby. CJ lost her baby – Finlay – in 2005. I told her about our Finley and she said she'd donate a small portion from the sale of each book to any charity we set up in his name. She's inspired me to make our own Finlay's Garden. Maybe at the cemetery so all the mums and dads have somewhere pleasant to go. I must buy a copy of the book. And one for the hospital.

We're going to arrange all the things for the Conway Suite into individual packs for parents. I've actually been into a baby shop today, looking at more stuff. I particularly like the soft blankets and tiny hats and socks they've got. I've found some great little cards for graves through eBay too. The seller agreed to let me have thirty for free so long as I bought one for myself. So I have.

It's starting to dawn on me quite how lucky we were with the aftercare we received in hospital, and the support we had from the funeral directors. Not everyone is as fortunate. Kim, Imogen's mum, told me they weren't even allowed to bathe Imogen, despite asking if they could. The skin on Imogen's cheek had peeled, so perhaps this was why. Kim told me that Imogen was induced because she'd died in the womb. Her skin may have deteriorated because of this. A baby's skin is fragile, of course. But I really do believe that parents should have the option to bathe their baby. The baby is dead and can't be harmed any more. The parents' wishes should be a priority. I don't see why a compromise couldn't have been agreed in Imogen's case. If it's really not possible to bathe the baby, then perhaps the parents can be supported while dabbing baby powder onto their baby's skin. They may be able to smooth the baby gently with cotton wool or a wipe. It simply isn't possible to overestimate the importance of this kind of ritual for a grieving parent. It was everything to me to be able to bathe Finley. I needed to do it. I am his mum. It was the only chance I had.

I promised myself I'd stop writing this journal once the post-mortem results arrive. That time is coming close. I can't believe I've made it this far. And I feel dismal that this process of writing might be coming to an end. I still have no idea how it will end. I don't want it to. I don't want to let go of this tiny piece of my son. Still, we haven't had the post-mortem results yet, so I don't have to stop writing. Not yet. After all this time, we still don't know what happened to Finley.

To Finley,

I never stop thinking of you. Every shop I go into, I see things for you. Soon your playground will be full of toys.

I have been hearing about lots of angel babies like you today – you will have even more friends to play with.

I love you a zillion times bigger than the sky, my darling baby boy.

Day 62

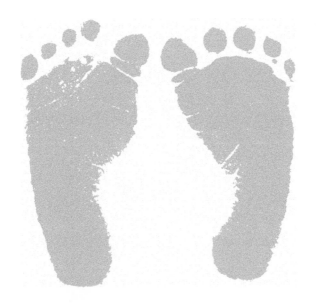

It's Finley's two-month Angelversary and all I've wanted to do is write. Angelversary is the name some of the other mums I speak to give to the date their babies died. So Finley would have been two months old today. He would have been smiling and holding his head up. There's a fair on, and we would've been taking him there to celebrate. We'd have bought him a balloon and tried to win a goldfish for him.

Instead, I've been at Finley's graveside. The caretaker has topped up the soil at last. Instead of playing with my baby, I've covered his grave with black binbags, straightened the border fence, fixed his toys and ornaments, and put some pebbles down around the edges. Bright blue stones. I've added large candles for more light and a ladybird solar light that Danni sent me. Lights are twinkling now on so many of the graves. It makes a pretty sight. To top it off, we've left Finley a wooden train from the fair that spells out F-I-N-L-E-Y. The train now marks his grave.

We met Katy and Roger at the fair with their daughter Ivy. Ivy persuaded me to take the teddy bear she'd won for Finley on the big wheel with me. So that he could see all the lights.

To Finley,

Happy two-month birthday little man. I love you so much and think of you every day.

I wish you were here with us, keeping us awake, smiling with a cute little grin that wrinkles your chubby cheeks. We could have been out for a walk along the canal or gone for a drive in the car today.

I hope you've enjoyed your day wherever you are.

Day 64

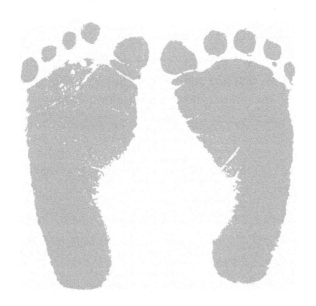

I don't feel I need to write so often these days. I'm much busier for a start. Or perhaps things are starting to get back to normal. I guess that's what people must think. But to be honest, there is no normal any more. Or if there is, I don't know what it is. Not yet. Things can't ever be the way they were again. And they can't be how we'd pictured them either. So, from now on, I guess we need to make a new normal.

I still find it hard to pick up the phone and call friends when I need them. And believe me I do need them. It's just, I guess, I don't really seem to know who I am. I mean, I've changed so much. In some ways, things feel more serene with me. Within me. My life has a real sense of perspective now. Small things don't worry me like they used to. And things that would never have bothered me previously now really irritate me. I don't have the patience I once did. People certainly found that one out in the post office today. There I was, waiting for a parcel, and they couldn't find it. I didn't hesitate. Just walked straight out.

I don't actually want things to get back to normal. Normal didn't always mean happy for me. I wasn't normally happy. It's time things changed. Things have already changed. No stopping that.

Writing every day before going to bed has been helpful beyond measure. All the thoughts, all the feelings – I've just been able to get them down onto paper. To get them out of my mind and stop worrying, stop listening to them. I'm sleeping better now too. Keeping busy helps.

To Finley,

I still think of you every day and wish you were here. I think of all the things we could do together.

You will always be a part of my life, but in a different way to what we'd imagined. We won't go to the park together; I won't watch you taking your first steps or chasing the cats.

Instead, I'll talk about you, write about you and teach people about you. You will be part of the lives of many people. We will remember you.

Day 66

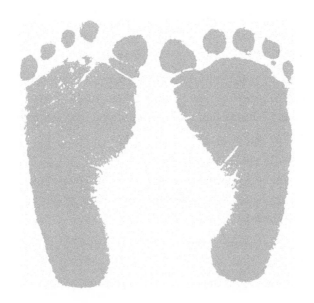

More time on Facebook and more mums who've lost babies. I've joined a group about pregnancy and baby loss awareness – it's Pregnancy and Baby Loss Awareness Week next week. The group has been discussing the International Wave Of Light event on Thursday. I wonder whether we could invite other people to join us at the cemetery. So I've been talking to Donna and Kim. If we run an ad in the local paper, anyone could turn up and it wouldn't be private. It might draw attention to the cemetery, and people might damage the graves. So we've decided to put notes on the other graves in the same section as ours. I hope no one finds this too intrusive. I know I wouldn't – I'd be touched to know people were thinking of us. And I'd hate to miss out.

To Finley,

We've left letters in their gardens for your angel friends' mums and dads. It'll be a special day on Thursday next week. We're going to light a candle for you, and send you a wish lantern. We'll light candles for some of your friends too. I hope you get to see how pretty it is from wherever you are.

Day 68

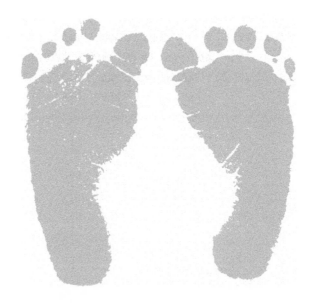

I've been busy organising a workshop for other parents like me. There needs to be more support, more guidance to help people feel better, to help them heal themselves. I'm lucky enough to have been able to support myself using techniques and approaches I've learned during the years I worked with therapists and on the self development courses I've attended. Now I can share what I know with others in circumstances similar to mine. I want to share it all.

Day 70

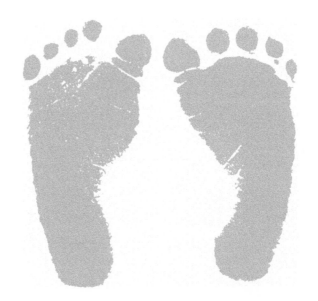

I'm in serious trouble today with Baz. I've crashed his car. If you tried to make it up you couldn't. I'd been to see Donna to talk about making gifts for the people coming to the workshop. I reversed down her driveway, my head full of foam butterflies and Christmas baubles with angel wings, my hands covered with dried glue and feathers. I stopped, changed gear and heard a crunch! It took me a while to grasp what I'd done – I'd reversed into a parked car. Seems I have issues with parked cars. And walls. They just ... um ... attract me.

The car needs a new bumper and back lights, so not too much damage done. Still, Baz was hardly smiling when I broke the news.

To Finley,

I thought you angels were supposed to look after us? You must have wanted a laugh today, at Mummy's expense.

Day 74

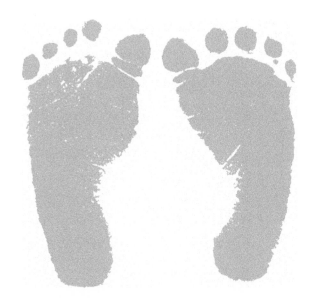

Any minute now there'll be two new babies in the family. I'll be an aunty twice over. Everyone will be excited. And Finley will be forgotten.

It's almost three months since Finley was born and I still can't quite grasp it. Time moves so fast. It helps that I've got all these events to focus on. There's the International Wave of Light and the Megan's World fundraiser for Cameron and Carter's headstone. But things aren't getting any easier. With the new babies due, it's all playing so heavily on my mind.

Ever since my godson was born, all I've wanted is to have a baby of my own. As we've watched him grow (and spoiled him no end), I've pictured what it would be like with my own. I've watched my friends and my cousins become parents, aunts and uncles. All these years, and now I'm going to be an aunty myself. Right when I don't think I can do it. I don't think I can be in the room with a newborn baby. I don't think I can hold my niece or nephew. Because it hurts so much. Physically hurts. When I go out, I see prams and babies everywhere I look. If I hear a baby cry, my body thinks it's my baby. I know it's not my baby. That my baby isn't here. But my body doesn't seem to know. Or care. How am I going to be able to hold my newborn niece and nephew when my body reacts like that?

To Finley,

I just want you to be here. I don't want to hold everyone else's baby. I want you here in my arms where you are supposed to be.

My body is here to look after you; I want to look after you. My arms automatically make your shape.

My hand is here to stroke your face. I can feel what it would be like to hold you and feel your breath on my neck as you snuggle in close.

I want to be able to smell your head and sigh over the new baby smell. I want to be the one discussing whether your eyes will change colour, or who you look like.

Instead, I have to wonder forever what colour eyes you have.

Day 77

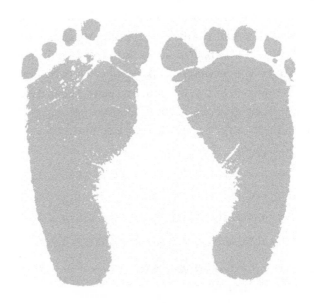

All around the world, people lit candles to commemorate International Pregnancy and Baby Loss Awareness Day. A wave of light lit up around the globe. It was a beautiful night. A peaceful celebration of Finley's life and the lives of all babies who are lost in pregnancy or after birth.

Before we left for the cemetery, I lit Finley's big candle, and spent a few minutes thinking about him. I don't know how much longer his candle will last. It's starting to collapse inwards and the name and photo stickers are peeling off. A friend called as we were getting ready. She needed some advice but I was abrupt and worry that I may have hurt her. Tonight is my night to be with Finley and that is all I can think about, I fumed. Then I hung up.

It surprised me to find at least thirty people at the cemetery. I hadn't expected Mum and Dad to turn up, but they did. Stephen and Denise didn't make it – their baby is due soon. I lit candles on Finley's grave and, as the sun was setting, placed tea lights on the other baby graves, giving special candles to Imogen, Joe, Cameron, Carter, and Jack. As the sun sank lower in the sky, the tea lights became more visible, glimmering along the lines of graves.

I handed out the wish lanterns. I'm so glad – it made the night extra special. It helped break the ice as people started chatting to each other trying to assemble their lanterns and work out how to light them. Luckily it stayed dry and there was only a gentle breeze. We set the lanterns off from the top of the hill. Looking down towards the graves, you could see all the candles and solar lights twinkling. Then, looking upwards, an amazing sight. Fifteen lanterns lifting off and gliding into the distance. The lanterns flew so high up in the sky that you could easily imagine angels reaching down from the clouds, catching them, or blowing them along.

Huddled around Imogen's grave, we ended the ceremony with readings. We included Raphael's poem from Finley's funeral, read by Donna's mum. It was very moving, and a huge success.

To Finley,

I have thought of you so much today. It's easy to imagine you sitting up among the clouds, looking down on a beautiful view.

As we sent your lantern up, I made a wish for you. I think I cheated a bit though, with a two-pronged wish. I wished for you to be back in my arms, so that we could cuddle you one last time. I added on the end: If that's not possible, I wish for you to be happy wherever you are.

Day 79

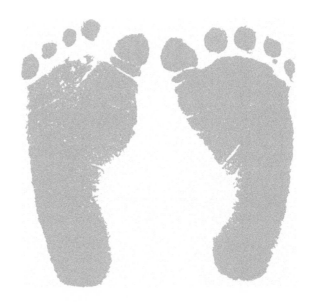

I can't sleep. I'm here alone in the dining room. Terrified. Stephen just texted to say that Denise has gone into labour and Robbie is on the way. I am worried about everything. I'm worried something will go wrong with the labour. I'm worried that Denise will be ill. Or that something is wrong with Robbie. I have no idea how my brother is going to manage the labour. I'm worried about whether or not I should go and see them in hospital. It's the same hospital where Finley was born and I don't think I ever want to go back there. I don't know how to tell my brother. Or if I can tell him that I do want to see them but am frightened I'll cry. I don't want to upset anyone.

Baz is worried about me and can't sleep either. He keeps coming downstairs to check on me. I reckon I may have been in denial, not really able to face the fact that I'm about to have a niece and a nephew. There was a time not so long ago when I was looking forward to this day so much I could barely contain my excitement. I was so eager for all our babies to play together and grow up together. It won't happen now and there's no justice in it. None at all.

To Finley,

Please look after Robbie and make sure he gets here safe and sound. We don't want any more heartache in this family. We need this baby to be well, smiling and happy. Help Denise and Stephen through the labour. I will never forget you baby boy, and I will make sure nobody else forgets you. Please help me find the strength to be an aunty instead of a mum.

Day 80

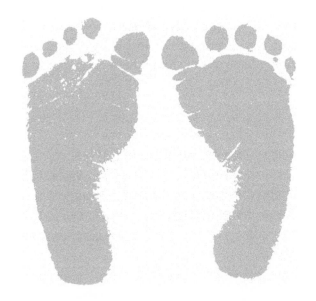

Robbie arrived at five fifty-two in the morning. Safe and sound. Stephen texted me to say Robbie was having breakfast. What a mixture of emotions I'm feeling right now. I'm jealous because Denise had exactly the kind of birth I had hoped for myself and visualised so often. She had the birth I had planned for. A short labour and a water birth using only a tens machine for pain relief. I doubt I'll ever get to have that dream birth. Even if I'm allowed a natural birth, it'll be induced and I'll be on a monitor the whole time.

I'm pretty angry at myself for being this jealous. Yet at the same time I feel delighted and relieved to know that Robbie is well. That he's here and he's healthy. I am shocked when I recall that five fifty-two was the exact time I'd had the scan of Finley that showed his last recorded heartbeat. That it's two months to the day today that we buried Finley. Everything makes me think of him now.

I made it to the hospital this afternoon. It took every bit of strength I had. Denise and Robbie were in the birthing centre where we'd been when my waters first broke. As soon as I arrived, Mum sat me down and handed Robbie to me. He is much smaller than Finley and makes snuffly noises. I cried as I held him. And when he opened his eyes, I was lost. I will never know what colour eyes Finley had. Finley never opened his eyes.

By the time Stephen gave Robbie his first bath, the tears were rolling down my face without stopping. I remember bathing Finley, but he was dead. He did not wriggle and he did not cry. This time round, leaving the hospital was no easier. It felt so wrong to be walking out of that same hospital again without a baby in my arms. It made no sense at all.

To Finley,

I miss you so much. This is unfair – you should be here with me. I shouldn't be upset that I have a nephew. I should be gazing into your eyes. And rocking you, not your cousin. I should be proudly showing people the videos of your first bath. This is not fair. I love you so much.

Day 82

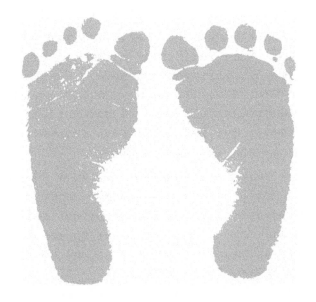

Amie went into labour last night and I couldn't sleep. The umbilical cord got wrapped around the baby's tummy. The baby went into distress and Amie had an emergency caesarean. Just as I had. But Amie's baby – Holly – arrived safe and well at eight thirty. I feel so mixed up about it. There was an identifiable reason for Holly to be distressed. The cord was wrapped round her. There was never any problem with Finley's cord, the staff had said. Holly weighed just five pounds six ounces. So much smaller than Finley. Without question, I would hate for anything to have happened to Holly. But I simply cannot make sense of the fact that she survived and Finley did not.

We'll go and see Holly on Wednesday. I'm nervous of course, but this time it's not the same hospital. I don't know whether I'm excited, anxious, fearful or all three. I don't know what I am. I'm afraid I'll cry, but that would hardly surprise anyone. In fact, I've always cried when I hold newborn babies. Even before we lost Finley. It's just such a moving experience. There really is something quite incredible about a creature so tiny coming into the world.

To Finley,

You have another cousin. A little girl. Someone you would have been able to look after.

You'd have grown up close, and you'd have been protective over her. In you, she would always have had someone to turn to.

Instead, I have someone else I need to visit who reminds me of what should have been. All those wasted dreams.

Day 84

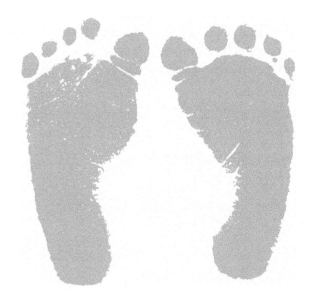

A different hospital, what seemed like a very long drive, and far too much nervous tension. This was something I wanted over and done with as soon as possible. And I felt absolutely awful for thinking that way about my new niece. Yet, despite my qualms, the hospital visit went well.

Amie was sore after her caesarean, but up and walking about. I don't think I've ever seen anyone as excited as Ed, in a shell-shocked kind of a way. He kept showing us Holly's hands, her tiny clothes. He's so much like Baz that I couldn't help thinking *This should be Baz. Baz should be showing off our baby's toes.* When Holly woke up, Ed changed her nappy. He's certainly going to need some practice at that! He got her feet all messy, ugh! So I showed him how to fold the nappy over while washing her, so that she stayed clean.

I had a superb, long cuddle with Holly and she fell asleep in my arms. She's tiny compared to Finley. She feels light to me and the wrong shape somehow. All the clothes Amie's parents had brought with them were too big for her. Amie's mum thought it was brave of me to be there at all. But facing this head on is the very best way for me to cope. Avoidance and denial make things harder in the long run. And you know what, I didn't feel quite as gloomy as I'd expected when I was cuddling Holly. It's going to get easier, I'm sure.

To Finley,

Your cousin is so cute. She is tiny – half the size you were. She needs so much looking after. I wish you were here to meet her.

I miss you so much. I would give anything – anything – to hold you in my arms and kiss your forehead again. I'd give anything for one more minute with you.

Holding other people's babies just makes me want you here. I love you so much I am going to burst.

Day 88

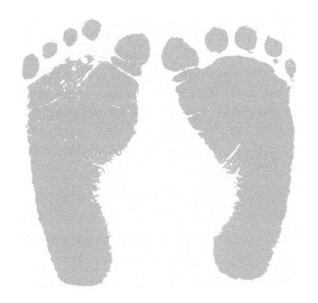

Heart-warming comments on Facebook have got me smiling again. I'd changed my status to: Tears again, silly eyes. A friend replied Leaky eyes are all part of being a yummy angel mummy. People will soon get used to it. Donna added Are your eyes broken too? Mine cry even when I'm not sad. I often wonder if the tears will ever stop. I sob at the smallest things. But I'm glad I can smile too.

To Finley,

You wouldn't want me to be sad would you?

Day 90

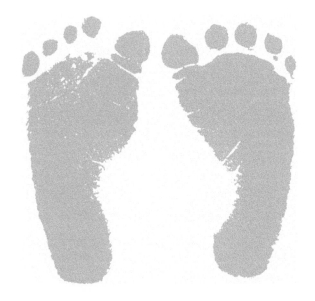

Bonfire night and we're just back from the local fireworks display. We go every year. After shutting the cats indoors and locking the cat flap, we take our little stroll up the road. This time last year I was just about to get a piece of news that would change my life forever. I can't help thinking back. Knowing that this year is different in a way I could never have foreseen.

I watched the fireworks surrounded by people with babies in pushchairs. I try so hard not to be jealous, but it's a struggle. It hurts to know that this should have been us.

Tonight, there was a mum yelling at her little boy. He'd climbed out of the pushchair, stood up in it and tipped it over backwards. It could have been really painful, and there she was, giving the poor kid a loud telling off. Thing is, she'd completely ignored his repeated requests to get out and be picked up so that he could see the fireworks. When I heard her shouting, it was all I could do to stop myself shouting back at her. I hate feeling this judgemental.

The fireworks were spectacular. Watching them, set against a huge gleaming moon made hazy by the clouds, I couldn't help but weep. And, as the fireworks flashed before that beautiful moon, I realised that Finley must have had a stunning view. It must be so different looking down on fireworks from above. Like looking down at the clouds when you're in a plane. My baby gets to see that every day.

> To Finley,
>
> It's warmed my heart today to imagine you and your friends sitting on the clouds watching the fireworks from above. I bet it looks so beautiful from up there. I hope you were wrapped up warm, and toasted marshmallows on the fire.

Day 96

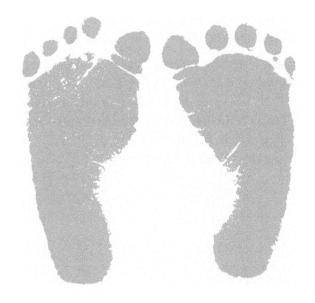

Visiting Finley's grave, it's clear that winter is on its way. The cemetery sits in a very open space on the side of a hill and is exposed to all the elements.

I've always enjoyed the changes of season in England. Watching all the different characteristics evolve. I can never decide which is my favourite. I love the autumn, all the leaves changing colour, their vibrant hues catching in the light and dusting the hills with cheer on sunny days. Winter snow and frost appeal to me too, although I'm less keen on the rain. This year, I'm especially looking forward to spring. I must plant more snowdrops and bluebells around the hawthorn tree by Finley's grave.

It was so windy overnight that Finley's teddy bear had blown over. I've made sure it's tucked under one of the pebbles that edge his grave now. Teddies from another grave have blown away too. It felt pretty grim, not knowing who they belonged to and not being able to put them back on the right grave.

To Finley,

I try and try to think of good things, lovely things, but sometimes it's too hard. We buried your body. I don't know if we made the right choice. As the winter is hurrying close, I think of you and whether you are frightened in the dark on your own, whether your feet are cold because I forgot your socks.

It was nice to see a blanket of leaves covering you, but how will it be to see the ground all muddy and sinking? What will it be like when your flowers freeze?

I try not to think of you being in the ground, but on cold dark days I can't help it. I'm sorry.

Day 100

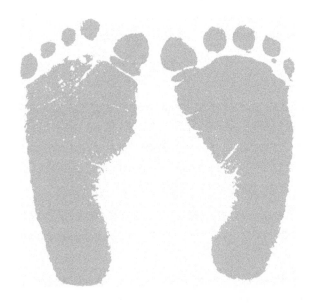

Twins Cameron and Carter were due to be born today. They grew their wings in July. They'd had twin-to-twin transfusion syndrome, and died after the surgery that had aimed to save their lives. Baz and I set some balloons off by the grave with their parents, Sherri and Dave. Sherri had attached message tags to the balloons. One was for Finley. The balloons got stuck in a tree on the other side of the road, where they remain even now. I wonder what the driver thought when the balloons narrowly missed his car.

There was a party for the twins at Sherri's afterwards. I gave her a card that said Congratulations on the birth of your twins, and inside wrote that they had grown beautiful wings. Sherri has set up a fantastic display on her kitchen sideboard. A large, sparkling angel stands right at the back. There are two teddies on either side, and Sherri added the two blue toy Beetles I'd given as gifts. On the angel's wings hang bracelets Sherri has made, and in front of it lies a bowl of pebbles and night lights burning in memory of the other babies Sherri has lost. She and Dave have lost eight babies altogether. Cameron and Carter actually share their due date with an earlier set of triplets. Sherri and Dave are blessed to have Kimberly, a beautiful two-year-old girl who was also one of twins. Kimberly gives us all hope and keeps us smiling.

Dotted around Sherri's display were small memorials for Joe, Finley and Imogen. For each baby, there's a card from Sherri, Dave and Kimberly. Lying beside the cards are black pebbles, each pebble with a letter painted in glitter on it spelling out the baby's name. There's a candle for each baby too.

In Finley's card, they'd written:

Please make sure you find Cameron and Carter and have a game of footie. I'm sure they will love that.

Please always be with your mummy and daddy. Let them know you are okay. Tell them you're their butterfly, their sunshine, even their smile.

Love you little man.

Sherri, Dave and Kimberly xxx

There's a photo of Finley in the display. How odd, Sherri found it in her cupboard. I've no idea how it got there. Perhaps he got inside some craft things I'd left there once. Still, Sherri made me laugh when she said it was just that Finley had wanted to come to the party early. Apparently, she'd tried to put his photo in several places, but it kept falling over. The only place it would stay put was with Cameron and Carter's photos. Later, I caught a glimpse of Baz blowing bubbles at the display and Sherri taking pictures of the bubbles as they blew in front of Finley's photo.

I'd promised Kimberly a bed time story, so I read her two books. She lay down, setting Finley's photo on her pillow. Walking down the stairs afterwards, I overheard Kimberly saying night night Finley. The tears welled up.

To Finley,

Did you hear the story I read? I wish I could read stories to you as we cuddle up under a blanket.

Day 103

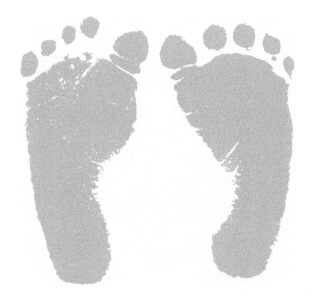

Out for coffee with Mum and I had to spend ages reassuring her that I really am doing okay. Certain people have been worrying her over the amount I'm talking about Finley on Facebook. I'm incensed. People only need to talk to me, to ask me how I'm feeling, and I'll explain! They certainly do not need to tell my family I'm grieving in the wrong way. It's outrageous.

So people reckon it's unusual for me to be speaking and writing about my son. And yet, for me, it would feel odd not to be. There have been strong comments about me displaying photos of Finley online too. Just because it may not be what people expect. Because people think they know what's right or wrong for me. Or because they can't handle it. It's my own personal decision what I do with my photos of my baby. This is uncharted territory. I've never experienced these emotions before. The grief, the sadness, the guilt, fear, pride and joy. The intensity of this love. All these things are new and powerful. I am a mum. I love my son. I am proud of him, and I think he is beautiful. It's my privilege to be able to share that with the world in the way I choose. Oh dear, I do hate trying to reassure Mum that everything's okay.

Just because I feel fine a lot of the time, that doesn't mean Finley isn't on my mind. Just as he would be if he were alive now. And, since he's often on my mind, I talk about him. It helps me when I talk about him. It helps me to remember that he was here. That we have a son. It helps me when other people talk about him too. I can't tell you if there'll come a time when I don't talk about him any more, or don't want to talk about him. Right now, I want and need to talk about my son. I love him and I miss him and he is still a very big part of my life. It's as natural as breathing in and out.

To Finley,

I love talking about you, writing about you – I even talk to you still as though you can hear me. This means you are still here, still close to me. Why don't other people understand this? How can they judge us? All I want is for you to be here with me.

Day 106

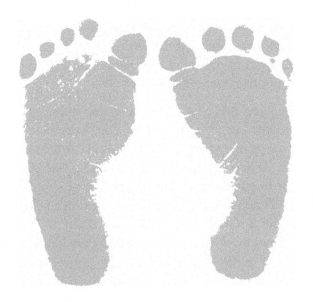

The pencil drawing I'd ordered a while back arrived in the post. It's by an artist who makes sketches from photos of stillborn babies. A friend had shown me the drawing of her baby and it was quite stunning. Her baby had been younger than Finley and had sore skin. But there was no sign of any discolouration in the sketch.

I saw the drawing of Finley and wept. Right there in the post office. It's hard to describe just how beautiful it is. Baz and I looked at it alongside the photo it was drawn from. It's a perfect replica but somehow softer. In both, Finley looks as though he is sleeping peacefully. The smooth lines of the pencil have enhanced the effect. Even the dimple on Finley's chin is there. But not the comma-shaped birthmark above his eyebrow.

The artist, Helen, had included a note alone with several copies of her drawing. It's been photocopied in blue, and the copies look gorgeous. We'll give one each to our mums, and get the postcard-sized print laminated so that it never gets ruined.

To Finley,

Sometimes when I haven't looked at your photograph for a little while I forget how beautiful you are. You truly are an angel, peacefully sleeping. The drawing of you just highlights how beautiful you are. I miss you so much that looking at you hurts.

Day 109

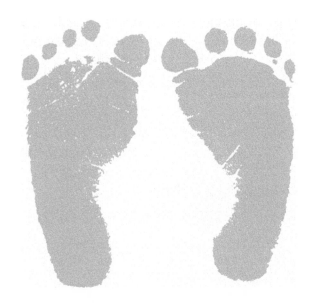

I keep bursting into tears. I just can't do this any more. I feel sick and I'm completely shattered. I have no energy left to fight with. Nothing.

It's a struggle just to get up in the mornings. I haven't showered, my hair is greasy and a mess. The doctor has taken some blood to check my iron levels. I mentioned to the nurse that we still haven't had Finley's post-mortem results back. So she's asked the doctor to chase them up.

I really, really don't want to hear the results. I'm terrified we'll discover that someone could have done something to save my baby. I can't stop worrying about it. I've only been managing so far by reassuring myself it was all an accident. Everything happened so quickly once they'd made the decision to do the emergency caesarean section. They couldn't have acted more quickly than they did.

But what if we find out that the caesarean should have been done when I first got to hospital? Or when I told the staff the meconium was thicker? Perhaps they should have acted when I first mentioned that the numbers on the monitor were dropping. What if they missed all those chances to save my baby? What if he didn't have to die after all? I know I should have fought harder for him. I knew something was wrong with the numbers.

They say Finley's case is next in the queue to be reported on. They've been feeding us that line since I first called up. Baz is getting so frustrated and angry that even he's been phoning now and he hates using the phone. I don't want the results. But I can't stop phoning either.

I am full of contradictions. I don't want the results but I need to know the results. I need to know what happened to my baby boy. But I don't want to find out that he died without cause or reason. Or out of negligence. What if someone made a mistake and it killed him? What if he could have been saved, where the hell will we go from there?

Apparently there's a shortage of pathologists in Bristol and some bodies have been sent to Oxford for post-mortems. I'm petrified that Finley could have been moved without our knowledge. Sure, we signed the post-mortem form. We gave the authorities licence to cut up our little boy. But I made sure at the time to explain to Finley where he was going and what would happen. I told him I was sorry he'd be hurt and messed about, but that we had no choice since we needed to know what had happened to him. I told him he would be close by to Nadine in the hospital in Bristol and that she would look after him. What if they moved Finley, or lost him; what if they got him muddled up with another baby? I can't stop thinking the worst. Thank goodness we had an open coffin and saw that it was our little boy in there, not someone else.

To Finley,

Soon we will find out what happened to you. I'll know if I did something wrong. I'll know if you were ill or in pain. I'll know what happened in those last moments you were alive. I'm so scared. What if we could have done something? What if there is a way you could have survived? I'm so sorry we failed you little man. We're supposed to look after you and keep you safe. We couldn't do this one little thing.

Day 110

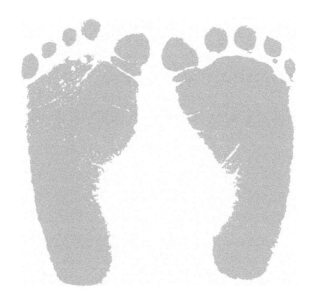

I feel like hell. I want to cancel today and move straight on to tomorrow. I've just had enough.

I did make it to Sherri's for a cup of tea. She's been busy making bracelets for our fundraiser night. She's so sweet, she's made one for Finley. It's lovely of course, but I'm going to struggle to fit it in his memory box.

People have been supportive on Facebook. But it's just one of those days. Someone told me to be strong for a little longer, or told us to be strong together. I just want to shout and scream at them all. Nothing anyone says to me today will be the right thing to say. I don't want to be strong. I want someone to wrap me up and put me away like a tortoise. I want to hibernate in a box in the airing cupboard until spring comes.

Day 111

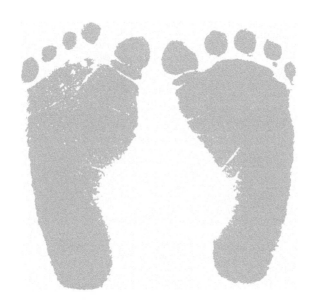

I still feel like hibernating. I managed to wash my hair. Just about. But then I couldn't be bothered to do anything with it. I just stuck a hat on, picked up some baggy trousers – which may or may not have been clean – and slung on any old top.

I'd arranged to meet Donna at the church for the meditation group. I went but couldn't concentrate. Sit still and relax? Come on!

Donna gave me a photo of a butterfly on the back of which she'd written a poem. A woman read it out at the meditation group. Although the poem made me cry, I'm so close to tears all the time these last few days that it was no surprise. It turns out that the woman who read the poem is a retired midwife. She actually made us give her a hug. Usually I'm happy to hug strangers. Say if I've been on an emotionally moving course and bonded with them. I give strangers hugs on Facebook all the time too. It's easy, you just type ((())). And sometimes you put the person's name inside the brackets for that personal touch. But I seriously did not want to hug this woman.

To Finley,

I have nothing to say. I can't find the words.

Day 112

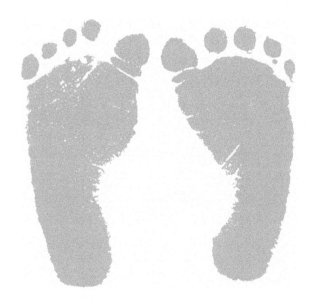

A real roller-coaster ride. Everything feels like it's rushing by at warp speed. I've had a call from the hospital. We're going to see a different doctor to get Finley's results. Tomorrow at midday.

I was with Sherri and Donna when I got the call. I've not been that wobbly since my niece and nephew were born and I think it gave them a bit of a shock. We all call a bad day a wobble, by the way. I'm so thankful that Dad's agreed to come with us. He'll be able to help us ask the questions we need to, if we find we can't do it ourselves. I want to use a tape recorder too so that I can concentrate and won't need to remember or write everything down.

I have to know what happened to Finley. It's not that I want to move on. That's not what I need. I will not be moving on from my son. Things may improve and become easier but I will not have moved on. I will not leave Finley behind. He is in everything I do. He is the reason I get up in the morning and he is the reason I live and love.

But, in order for me to live, I choose to know what happened to my son. I have to find out. I feel peaceful knowing that I am making this choice. I don't have to do it. I could choose to carry on with life as it is. I could continue to believe that it was an accident and that nobody could have prevented it.

It's late at night now. It's the windiest night I can remember in a long time. At the cemetery, fences have blown over and it looks as if half a tree is on Finley's bed. Kim would go crazy if she saw all the leaves. But I find them quite soothing. I've always loved walking in the woods, scrunching leaves underfoot. And it looks just as if Finley has made a magical quilt out of the leaves to keep himself warm. Even so, I did move the branches away. Why on earth I thought night-lights would stay lit in gale force winds, I don't know. I couldn't even light the wick. I got upset thinking that would mean Finley was in the dark. I sat on his tree trunk sobbing. The light had been so dull all day that even his solar lights weren't working. Yet I could hear his wind chimes ringing clearly through the gusts.

I've been talking to two close friends and they've helped me feel better about tomorrow. Fraser even dared to say I was being a little self-indulgent. Trust Fraser. He's right, and I laughed – this is self-indulgent. I get it. There's definitely something to be said for indulging the tears when they're there ready to fall. I want to cry. I want to feel this pain. I am connected to Finley in peace, love and joy, but also through my anger and pain. The pain is useful. It will help me focus tomorrow and get the answers I need. If I go into the meeting in a state of total acceptance, I mightn't get any answers. So, I've even been listening to Finley's songs on my mp3 player, deliberately listening to all the ones that make be cry. At the cemetery, I sat on the tree trunk at the side of his grave and listened to a woman sing about a cradle of wings and I sobbed my heart out. I stayed on until I got too cold and spooked out by the shadows.

So I've spent most of the night talking to people on Facebook. Usually I get pretty easily carried away, spotting the word angel everywhere I look. On a different day, or if I were slightly less cynical, I'd take these as messages from Finley. Today that's a step too far.

Someone with Angel in their name has posted a status update saying: Rejoice in the small miracles of your life, everyday. Allow your light to shine. When you begin to see and to feel this light shine within you, you will know that what you are doing is completing your journey; one day at a time. Today this makes me want to scream. I have no light. It has disappeared. My spirit has been hit by the credit crunch. Completing my journey, nope I'm not doing that. What a crock. Tomorrow I'll find out what stopped my son's journey before it had even started.

I just don't know. Do I want a reason or not? My baby is in the ground. In a box a bit harder than a shoe box and a tiny bit bigger. Buried in the ground. Why is a nine pound seven ounce baby in the ground and not in my arms?

If someone is responsible, what can I do? I can't exactly thwack the damned doctor can I? Although Dad might. I'm just going to crumple, I know it. What if no one's responsible? Will that be better? Will it be easier to take it if there's a medical reason? An infection? Or will that mean it was my fault, my body's fault?

And if they haven't found a reason, what then? What happens when I get pregnant again if we don't know why Finley died? How will we get through all those weeks of another pregnancy not knowing whether or not the same thing will happen again? This shouldn't even happen once. Yet in the UK it still happens to seventeen babies every single day. The statistics are all too clear to me now. They're stuck in my head. And I don't want to know. There were twelve deaths just like Finley's in the same hospital in a single month. If that doctor tomorrow tells me this is rare (he said that to Donna), I think I might scream.

There's more and it's worse. We'll be meeting the doctor in the maternity unit. I'd forgotten that until now. The same maternity unit where we spent those precious days after Finley was born. The same ward Baz and I had stepped into, excited and nervous, ready to meet our new baby. When we staggered out, we were devastated. We'd left our baby wrapped in a blanket in a cot in a strange room with a virtual stranger. She may have been a plain-clothed saint, but we'd only met her that morning. When we left, I was hugging a feathered pillow, fat and squishy but not baby-shaped. A pillow, not my baby. Since that day, I've been back once, to visit my newborn nephew. And now we have to return to hear what happened to Finley. How can that be right? Where is the consideration? The compassion? Do these people not understand what this is like for us? Do they not care?

We'll wait in the maternity reception for the doctor to come and get us. In front of us, there'll be pregnant women attending scans, full of excitement. Behind us, the labour ward will be full of screaming babies and women yelling out with labour pains. I remember screaming. But not for that reason. I was screaming a grief-stricken No! when I'd found out my baby was dead.

I have a list of questions. But I don't want them answered. I want to show the doctor my photo album. I want him to see my beautiful baby boy, and I want him to look closely at the photos. I want him to see what has been lost. I want him to see what his words cannot return. I want him to see that.

Day 113

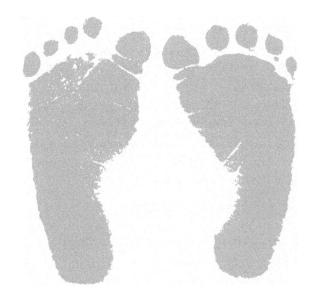

Well that's it. Over and done with. At noon, we had an appointment with the consultant to find out what had happened to Finley. An ordeal that lasted an excruciating two-and-a-half hours. We arrived early and reported to the midwife in the maternity unit. We had to suffer the indignity of hearing our son's post-mortem results in the very maternity unit where we'd gone to give birth to him such a short time ago. Astounding.

We sat in the waiting area by the coffee machine right at the centre of the reception and in full view of everyone. Last time we sat here, I was seven months pregnant and we were awaiting a tour of the birthing unit. Today, as we waited to hear why our son had died, I counted three softly-lit black-and-white posters of bare-chested fathers clasping their babies. I also was forced to witness four pregnancy bumps of various sizes, two babies, two babies' cries and one father discussing his partner's progressing labour at the top of his voice. One of these days I will give in to the urge to shout out in a public place My baby died! Do you have any idea how hard it is for me to see you? Not today.

The insensitive treatment continued. The secretary took us down a corridor past the expressing room and into an office. On the office wall, a bookcase was littered with brochures called things like Saving Lives, all of them covered in photos of cute little baby hands and feet. I lost count of the number of babies I heard crying. I swear we must have been on the postnatal ward. How could I possibly concentrate on what this man was saying about my baby, with the noise of all these healthy live babies crying outside. My stomach still flip flops every time I hear a baby cry. Will that ever stop?

Against the odds, I found the strength to ask what I needed to ask. I showed the consultant my photo album. I insisted he call Finley by his name. Finley is a human being and not a clinical case.

It's over now and I cannot honestly say that I am any the wiser. We haven't even had the full copy of the post-mortem results. The pathologist wanted some answers from us about AT before finalising his report. And the consultant wouldn't give me a copy of the preliminary report he was reading from. Truly incredible. Surely the pathologist gives the answers not the parents?

We now know several things that did not kill Finley. We have no conclusive answer as to what did. Finley had meconium in his lungs. But this did not kill him as he didn't take a breath. There was bacteria in his stomach. But this did not kill him. It was most likely to have been introduced when the doctors attempted to resuscitate him, or from the umbilical cord. Blood tests showed I had marginally low thyroxine, but this did not kill Finley. Tests also showed that Finley had low oxygen levels, which probably stopped his heart. The specialists don't know what caused the low oxygen levels, and could say nothing about when this problem occurred.

The consultant hadn't known that Finley was the twelfth baby to use the Conway Suite that month. He told us that six in every one thousand births end in stillbirth and that there is a total of three thousand births at the hospital each year. I was impressed with my mental arithmetic under pressure, calculating that this makes an average of eighteen stillbirths a year. I was getting angry, saying that this would mean one to two each month. But there are three babies buried in Finley's cemetery who died at full term, from the start of July until the start of August. The consultant promised he would investigate the numbers of stillbirths in this period and get back to me.[iii]

I'm glad I'd had the foresight to record the meeting, as I didn't take it all in. The consultant talked us through everything that had happened during my pregnancy, all the test results, the labour and my postnatal care. I missed a lot of the detail. I was distracted as soon as I heard him say that they hadn't acted immediately because I was distressed and needed time for the information to sink in. Time to get used to the idea that this birth couldn't be everything I'd wanted. I took this to mean that I was at fault. I hadn't agreed to the induction straight away. But I don't think it was made very clear to me what was going on. No one told me I could lose my baby. I had to ask: would it have made any difference if I had been induced? If I had not been so determined to have a natural birth, and anxious about being induced; if I had requested an induction straight away, would Finley be alive now?

Other points stand out in my memory and will probably haunt me. Apparently, policy does not advocate caesarean section when a woman presents with meconium in her waters in early labour.[iv]

Recommendations are to examine the quality of the meconium and to consider continuous monitoring. In my case, the midwives had given differing suggestions early on, and did not monitor me continuously. In an ideal world, the consultant told me, I would have had one-to-one care and been admitted to the labour ward. But it was too full that night.

Thank goodness for Dad. He was more detached than I could be and kept repeating the question: Would Finley be alive if he had been delivered earlier? Yes, the consultant said. He would be alive. But it would have been very unlikely for a caesarean to have been done any earlier, because Finley's heartbeat was strong for much of the night.

I don't know where any of this knowledge leaves us. There is no indication that anything like this will happen in a subsequent pregnancy. That's a relief. But it shouldn't have happened this time either. Had someone made an assertive decision even ten minutes earlier than they did, my baby would now be sitting up, gurgling and smiling at me. I don't know where to go from here.

Our son is dead. Our baby is gone. He is not here where we can see him and care for him. We miss him and think about him every day. We cannot have the one thing we long for. There will always be something missing.

It's time for bed. It's two in the morning and I am beyond exhaustion. I only had a few hours' sleep last night. Perhaps I ate something earlier, I'm not sure. My eyes are swollen and I am cold and shivering.

It feels like I've been flattened by a steam roller. How can I get back up after this? Which way is up?

Hibernating like that tortoise sounds about right.

Epilogue

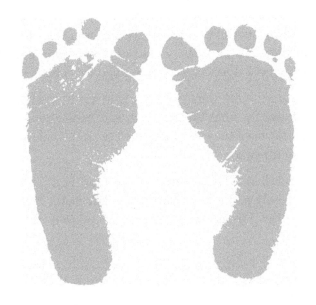

Dear Finley,

Over a year has passed since we met you and said our goodbyes to you. A great deal has happened in that time. I have everything to thank you for and such a lot to tell you. I can just imagine you growing up. You'd be walking now; I know you'd be cheeky and mischievous, wanting to know what everything is. I might even have tidied up the house to make it safe for you to run around in. I can almost see your chubby little cheeks and your curly hair.

We went away to Tenerife at Christmas time, but didn't forget about you. We took your photo with us, and sent you up a lantern from the beach on Christmas day. We thought of you as we went on a boat ride to see the dolphins. I got seasick so stayed out on deck when the sun started to set. Everyone else went inside. All of a sudden, a pod of dolphins leapt up just ahead of the boat, and I turned to watch them play in the waves as we passed. It was the perfect picture of freedom, all those dolphins cavorting through the waves just as the sunset was turning the sea fantastic shades of red and gold. I imagine you to be that free. Only ever surrounded by beauty.

Going away must have helped us, because something special happened just after we got back home. We found out that we will be having another baby.

For your first birthday, we tidied up your special resting place, and cleaned all the blue stones. You got lots of presents and cards, so we opened them with you. Nana and Grandad came along, and we sent a bunch of balloons up to you. I gave you some flowers in the shape of a number one. I'm sorry the grass had overgrown. I feel guilty that I haven't been to see you for such a long time. I got too upset for a while. It was so hard knowing I had your sister inside me, and that she won't know you.

A few weeks after your birthday, you became a big brother. I know you were looking after us, and made sure your sister Toni-Joi arrived in this world safe and sound. She was a bit poorly and had to stay in hospital at first. I was really frightened for her. But she's getting big now. When Daddy and I look at her, we feel happy that she is with us, but so very sad that you're not here too. She looks so much like you, Finley. This week she was weighed and measured and now that she's six weeks old, she weighs the same as you. When she is sleeping in my arms I think of you there too. I remember how it felt to hold you and how I longed to feel your breath on my cheek.

I hope you look in on us from time to time. But please don't keep your sister awake at night.

You are my son. You are my light, my love and my inspiration. I always refer to you as my little boy. But you are not little. You have a soul a zillion times bigger than the sky. You have reached out and touched more people than we could imagine. People your daddy and I know well, your family and our friends. But you've also touched the lives of many people we've never met.

In choosing us as your parents, and this time to arrive, you have blessed this corner of the world. You are responsible for helping numerous people to reflect on their life with gratitude. Your time here was short, but ever so precious, and you have brought about changes on a grand scale. Your daddy and I will enjoy our lives, we will enjoy this moment right now because it is all too soon over. I sometimes think I wish things were different. But I am also thankful for the way things are. I would always choose to have you Finley. We are treasured to have known you, honoured to have held you and blessed to be able to continue your story. I like to think that you have another important job to do, and that someday I will hear all about your adventures.

You have created more love than I ever thought possible. I love you so much more than possibility allows. In knowing you, I have found a love I didn't know could exist and that is truly a zillion times bigger than the sky. I have discovered peace, joy and happiness. In knowing you I have discovered myself.

With lots of love to you my darling baby boy. Much Loved. Always Remembered.

Mummy.

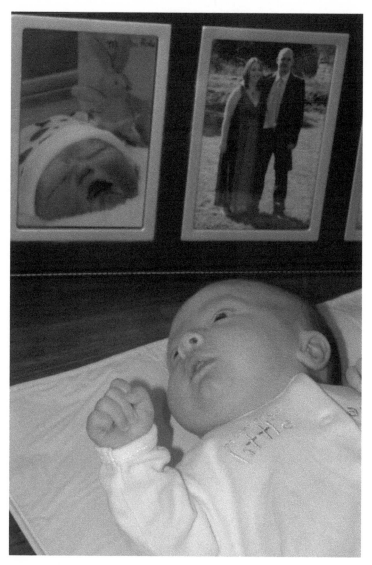

Family portrait. Five-week-old Toni-Joi looks at photos of Finley, Baz and me.

Dear Parent

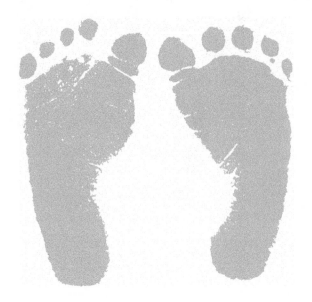

I am so very sorry that we meet like this. Whether you have recently left your angel in the hospital, or whether it's some time since your baby grew wings and flew from your arms, my thoughts are with you. I am sorry for your loss. If you are at the beginning of your journey, then when you are ready to reach out, please know that there is a wealth of information and advice out there to help you as you take your first steps. Please start by visiting www.finleysfootprints.com. I would also like to thank you in advance for the amazing difference the little life you brought into this world will make. In his short time in our arms, Finley made a profound difference to the lives of our family, our friends, and many people we didn't even know. For such a little guy, he made one huge impact.

I urge you to reach out, because there are many other mums and dads who are holding their hands out to you, willing and able to help. We all blow kisses to our little angels every night, but who knows where they go? Maybe some are caught by your little one as they smile down at you, catching the diamonds as they fall from your eyes.

I hope you've found some comfort following our journey and that reading about our experiences helps you find the strength to survive your own. You may not believe me now, as I couldn't believe myself not so long ago, but things do get easier, and in the right ways. There have been hurdles to overcome greater than we could have imagined, but we have survived. I can now acknowledge the joy I feel at having known Finley. I am blessed to have had the opportunity to learn the lessons he was here to give us. Perhaps his soul chose to come in order to show us the extent of love it is possible to have for another little person. Perhaps he came to show us that the world is full of an incredible love, a love that we often feel so much more easily before we're born and after our bodies die.

We cannot help but wish that things were different – for us and for you. But all we can do is make the most of where we are today in this moment. This is a huge lesson to learn and it can change your life. As it did mine. Life is short. Sometimes so very short that it is barely even a life. However, I have learnt that even though Finley did not have a heartbeat outside of my body, he was alive. Even though he no longer has a shell here on this earth, he is alive. He is in every step I take, every word I write, every conversation I have, every flower I see, every cloud that floats by, and in every butterfly and every rainbow. Your angel is too.

I wrote my story of life after Finley to honour his memory and to keep him alive. This book started as a way to keep myself sane in the very dark days after Finley was born. I found that it helped me to write down the mess of thoughts that were chattering away incessantly in my head. Once I'd written my thoughts down, they stopped moving so fast and seemed less frightening, less overwhelming. Writing helped me achieve some degree of order out of chaos. Having put my story on paper, I feel happy. Happy that now I have one more very special item to keep in the memory box in Finley's room.

I find now that I stand in a world of possibility and opportunity. For there is no longer any fear. I would really love all the mums and dads who have lost children at any stage of pregnancy or childhood to know that there is nothing to fear. For if our soul has chosen this path before we arrive here, then we owe it to ourselves to learn the lessons placed in front of us. We are special people, to be parents to such special babies. And if our babies live on, then truly we never die. And if we never die, then anything is possible.

Follow your heart. Follow that little voice that tells you you can.

Listen to that voice – it is your own special angel.

Always with you celebrating everything you do.

Dear Professional

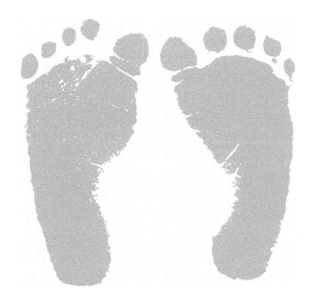

If you work with parents who have lost a baby (to miscarriage, stillbirth or other medical complications), then you have a very special job. You are in the privileged position of being able to help these people through the early days of a profoundly traumatic experience which will change their lives beyond recognition. In fact, you are in the very best position to assist in making this experience less traumatic. Your job is to guide these distraught parents, who will be in a state of shock, through the process of creating lasting memories of their baby. You may find that you come up against your own fears, uncertainties or judgments in the process. But you can be certain that if you do this one thing for these parents, your actions will make all the difference. Just as, in the book, the wonderful memories of Finley that we were so fortunate to have had the chance to make, changed everything.

I hope I have made it clear in this book that we hold all the professionals we encountered during those first months in the highest esteem. We have only the deepest respect and gratitude for the midwives, the vicar, funeral directors and other healthcare professionals who supported us. It is because of them that we have many, many treasured memories of our little boy. We would not have memories of him if it hadn't been for these people making the suggestions they did, and sometimes quite firmly. We were in such shock at the time and incapable of thinking of any such ideas ourselves. We needed to be led through our options steadily, a little at a time, sometimes repeatedly. Under the stress of a recent loss like ours, even the simplest decision feels impossible to make. We were so consumed by the horror of it all that the list of things we needed to consider, act on or decide in a single moment was more than we could manage alone.

I firmly believe that one of the reasons I am surviving this experience in the way I am is because we were able to spend three days in hospital with Finley after he died. Over the course of those three days, and with the professional support I received, I was gradually able to come to terms with Finley's death. For a range of different reasons, most parents in my position do not have this opportunity. It is my conviction that more time and the proper assistance are vital before a parent can fully accept that their baby has died. Had we left hospital on the first day, I would never have bathed my son, changed his nappy, dressed him in smart clothes, spent the night cuddling him or read him a bedtime story. We would never have had the chance to video these events. I would never have been able to hold all those outfits when I got home. We would have had no 'happy' memories of our baby, and no opportunity to express the natural parental instincts we felt when he was born.

I am eternally grateful to Jill, the wonderful midwife who managed to make it clear to us that we had just that one opportunity to make our memories. This is perhaps the most important message healthcare practitioners can convey to parents in circumstances like ours. Acknowledging the baby as a baby is a vital part of coming to terms with baby loss. Creating memories is a key step in the process. As is the ability to acknowledge and express any natural parental instincts without stigma. There is only this moment, there is only today. There will not be a tomorrow, there will not be a lifetime of memories. There is just this short space of time between the baby's birth/death and the funeral for the parents to hug, kiss and physically care for that baby. People always told us they couldn't imagine doing all the things we did with Finley. That it took guts. But the real reason we have the photos, videos, mementos – all these memories – is that we didn't want to have any regrets. We didn't want to regret not having done everything we could do with our baby while we could.

As professionals working in this field, you have the responsibility to inform parents of their options. I would urge you to make sure that you and your team are well versed in every option available in order that you can share this knowledge with the parents in your care, make suggestions sensitively and support parents' choices to the best of your ability. As I explained in my story, a friend who lost her baby at term was told she was unable to bathe the baby, and so never had the opportunity. Now she has to live with the guilt and regret. We still don't know whether or not she was given the correct information. If she was, she should have been told why this choice was ill-advised. She should have been able to make an informed decision or else offered an alternative.

I will always be thankful that someone asked me that one question What do you want your last memory of your baby to be?

I couldn't have known how vital that memory would become in the months that followed. I can't express how relieved I am that we lay our baby down to sleep, left him in a cosy room and asked a midwife to stay with him so he was not alone. I may have wanted to hand my baby over to the people at the morgue myself and ask them to look after him as if he was alive; I may have requested someone to carry him to the door to wave goodbye to us; or asked for him to be taken out first so I didn't have to walk away from him. So many choices for that single moment. But because we had the choice, we did it in the way we wanted to and so we have no regrets. By valuing this vital part of the healing process, you can ensure that no parent in your care ever has to have any regrets either.

Please do not let your own fears or feelings limit you. As you read in my story, people often reacted strongly to our choices. Clearly, there are all kinds of fears and taboos surrounding what we did. You are the very people best positioned to help remove these. Parents need to know that their instincts are acceptable. That there's no shame in wanting to wash or dress their baby, cuddle and kiss him or her. They need to know that they can't hurt their baby by doing these things. They need to know that no one can hurt their baby now and that the baby is no longer feeling any pain.

Because we were warned that Finley's nose may bleed when we moved him and that his bowels would leak, it was not so much of a shock when these things happened. In fact, I felt good being able to clean him up because it meant I had cared for my baby. I took off his nappy to give him a bath, and for an instant it was like having a baby who was alive. Rather than suppressing them for fear or shame, this allowed me to express the powerful maternal instincts I was feeling.

I felt frightened so much of the time. Frightened of everything. I am thankful that people took the time to take that fear away from me. As soon as I was given all the information about something, the fear dissolved. I was terrified of the post-mortem in case it hurt Finley. I was anxious about seeing him afterwards because of what he would look like. People took the time to explain what would happen and what I could expect, and suddenly it didn't frighten me any more. That's all it took – time and a little compassion. Because my fear was diminished, I was then able to have my wish and see my baby one last time, bring him home and let him sleep one night in his cot. I could talk to him, and most of all I could see that he was not a monster. He was a baby, my baby, and he was cosy and sleeping. Then all I had to worry about was the fact he had no socks on!

My own experience was life-saving precisely because we were given all the options and allowed to make our own informed decision based on comprehensive information. For instance, while we were told we could keep Finley in the room with us if we wished, the recommendation was that he be kept in the morgue overnight because otherwise his skin would deteriorate. We chose to keep Finley with us. The thought of Finley being with strangers was more upsetting to us than the thought of his skin worsening. I was even able to hold him throughout the night on our last night together. His skin did change – his lips got darker. But overall the skin colour became much more even. He actually looked better after three days than he had on the day he was born. If a hospital has a cold cot of course, things become far easier on parents who have to make such choices. A cold cot ensures that the baby deteriorates less quickly and so can remain with the parents as long they wish. In an ideal world, I would like to see hospitals able to loan parents a cold cot so that they can take their baby home for the desired period of time.

All this said, the most important factor in our survival was time. The length of time we spent in hospital. The time people took with us to make sure we understood all the information and had considered our decision. As much time as we needed, not as much time as the pressures of the job would allow. Jill's care was above and beyond the call of duty – she stayed with us well after the end of her shift. The experience of grief is an individual one. But the right information delivered with time and compassion is indispensable in every single case.

I hope I have shown in my own story that, while this is a traumatic experience, a lot of good can come out of it. The things you tell parents in your meetings with them will have a huge influence in this respect. If you inform a parent that this is the most traumatic experience they will ever have, your perspective will dominate the experience of their grief. If you advise them that they will be miserable and shocked, then these are the aspects of their experience they will be most likely to focus their attention on. There is another way. It is possible for you to help make this a beautiful experience that will bring peace and be full of love. You can make that difference. You can be part of the process that transforms giving birth and becoming parents to an 'angel baby' from an experience of trauma and loss to one of beauty, stillness and love. You can help remove the fear, anger and some of the pain simply by giving your time, compassion and human understanding. Let me say this one more time: You can make the experience of giving birth and becoming parents to an 'angel baby' beautiful, peaceful and full of love.

You will find information about dealing with baby loss, and the different options available, at www.finleysfootprints.com. Details of hospital packs and our cold cot campaign can be found at www.towards-tomorrow.com.

Afterword

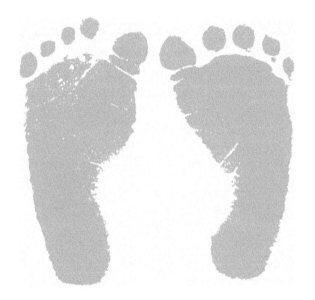

As you may have noticed, during the months following Finley's birth I frequently reflected on the experiences of other parents who lose a baby. Are they likely to receive the same kind of care as us? Be given the same choices in and out of hospital? Will they be supported in the most beneficial way possible by medical teams, friends and family, and others responsible for their care? What access do they have to information and services that may help alleviate their suffering? In fact, a large part of my journey after Finley has been to look carefully at what type and range of support is on offer for other parents like us, and to draw from my own experiences to design services capable of helping meet their needs.

As a result, the time since Finley's birth has also seen the birth of two wonderful organisations, Finley's Footprints and Towards Tomorrow Together.

Finley's Footprints is an information resource and support service for parents, allied professionals (e.g. midwives, funeral directors and health visitors) and charitable organisations involved with the care of bereaved parents and families, or those of terminally ill children. We aim to improve the consistency of care parents receive following baby loss. In particular, we work to improve the confidence of the professionals who provide parents with support; to enable charities to undertake their own support services as effectively as possible; and to assist parents in establishing some degree of control over their experiences as well as in discovering a sense of peace in the midst of their sadness.

Our range of services specifically for health and allied professionals and charities include online resources and training materials; coaching, training, workshops and inspirational talks. For parents, we provide online semi-structured coaching groups; a full range of useful resources; a strong social networking presence; individual coaching; workshops and international events. We also make available products such as books, and our annual conference brings parents, professionals and charities together to develop a shared knowledge and understanding. You can find us on the web at www.finleysfootprints.com.

Towards Tomorrow Together raises funds to support parents who have lost a baby or a child at any age or stage of pregnancy with the aim of helping those bereaved parents take their first tentative steps towards tomorrow.

Our charitable fundraising activities currently support three projects:

1. Acknowledgement packs distributed to hospitals, hospices and individuals. Each pack contains a selection of items specifically chosen to help parents through the first few days after their baby is born, enabling them to create vital memories, and encouraging them to express natural parental instincts.

2. Cold cots/cooling plates supplied to hospital maternity units for use in cases of baby loss.

3. A financial assistance fund available to finance emotional support for parents any time after a loss. Applications are considered from parents requiring services such as complementary therapies, coaching and workshops.

You can support Towards Tomorrow Together by donating via the website at www.towards-tomorrow.com or by emailing mel@towards-tomorrow.com.

Acknowledgements

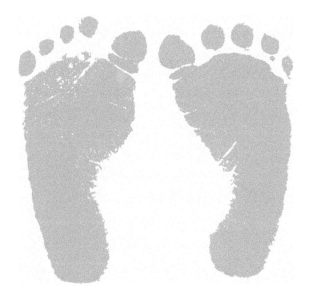

There are so many people to thank. My special thanks go to some very precious babies who captured my heart: Cameron, Carter, Joe, and Imogen. Thanks also to Norma, who patiently read and edited the very first draft of the book. Norma worked hard to teach me various points of English grammar including how to use a semicolon (which I still don't understand!). Thank you to Isabel for accepting my rather random initial questions about how to write a book and for all those midnight phone calls. When she first asked to see a few sample chapters, I replied I can't, my book doesn't have chapters! But for some reason, Isabel saw a diamond in the rough and supported me through the process of letting go of Finley and allowing the book to take shape.

Thank you to all my friends and family: there are too many of you to mention individually here. Every single one of you has helped me take an important step on my journey. I know you haven't always known what to say or what to do, but being there was enough.

Latterly, thank you to Jenny for her wonderful understanding of Finley and her beautiful artwork. My thanks also to Suzy for her ability to complete the project and finish the book.

Finally, thank you to Dr Baz, my husband. Baz has for the most part been exceptionally patient while my head has been buried in my laptop. Baz's love, comfort and humour – which he maintained, despite being needle phobic, when giving me injections – have got me through the long hard days.

[i]As this is a true story, the names of the people (and some of the places) involved have been changed to protect their identity. However, I have retained my own name as well as the names of my husband and son. Where parents have made a special request that I include the real name of their baby, I have done so.

[ii]Where hospitals ensure that cremation takes place at the end of the day, the baby's ashes may be received.

[iii]We have since received a letter from the consultant confirming that there were five stillbirths in the period from June through August. We assume that the figures we were given of twelve stillbirths in one month include all births from sixteen weeks onwards. A birth is only classified as a stillbirth after twenty-four weeks. The consultant gives no detail in his letter of what criteria were used to calculate the statistics.

[iv]'Intrapartum Care: Care of healthy women and their babies during childbirth', NICE clinical guideline 55 (Sep 2007), p. 42. Available at:

www.nice.org.uk/nicemedia/pdf/IPCNICEGuidance.pdf

Lightning Source UK Ltd.
Milton Keynes UK
UKHW01f1431041018
329938UK00001B/65/P